INFECTION CONTROL

The British Medical Association Guide

Published on behalf of the British Medical Association by

Edward Arnold

A division of Hodder & Stoughton

LONDON   MELBOURNE   AUCKLAND

INFECTION CONTROL

A report from the BMA Professional and
Scientific Division.

Project Director: Dr John Dawson
Written by: Dr Michael Henderson
Editor: David Morgan
Editorial
Secretariat: Audrey Porter
Tara Lamont
Hilary Glanville

Illustrations: Taurus Graphics

© 1989 British Medical Association

First published in Great Britain 1989

British Library Cataloguing in Publication Data

Infection control.
1. Man. Communicable diseases. Control
I. British Medical Association, *Board of
Science and Education*
616.9'045

ISBN 0-340-49655-X

Typeset in 10/11pt Paladium by Colset Private Limited,
Singapore.
Printed and bound in Hong Kong for Edward Arnold, the
educational, academic and medical publishing division of
Hodder and Stoughton Limited, 41 Bedford Square, London
WC1B 3DQ by Colourcraft Ltd.

Acknowledgements

Thanks are due to the following copyright owners for
permission to reproduce their photographs.

Barnaby's Picture Library: 1a, b, 2, 4, 5, 28, 57, 59,
77
BMA News Review: 55, 64, 65
Central Electricity Generating Board: 10 (patient), 14
**Electron Microscopy Unit, London School of Hygiene
and Tropical Medicine:** 20b, 22b, 25a, b, c, d, 26b
Mr Mark Edwards, London: 38
**Dr David Evans, London School of Hygiene and
Tropical Medicine:** 31 (tsetse fly), 32a, 78
**Dr David Hockley, National Institute of Biological
Standards and Control:** 23c
Ms Jane Jones: 31 (wild pigs)
Dr Q N Karim, St Mary's Hospital: 51a, b
**Dr Richard Lane, London School of Hygiene and
Tropical Medicine:** 10 (flea), 32c, 56
Dr Christopher Lee, Bristol: 34a, b, 35a, b, 37a, 39
**Dr Sebastian Lucus, University College Medical
School, London:** 42
Mr David Morgan, BMA: 23a, b
Dr Vivienne Nathanson, BMA: 74, 81
**Mr Lennart Nilsson, Boehringer Ingelheim INT
GMBH, Bonn:** 54b
Rex Features: 6
Mr Steve Richards: 27, 62a, b, 70
**Audio Visual Dept, St Mary's Hospital Medical
School, London:** 40b
Salvation Army International Heritage Centre: 50
Science Photo Library, London: 30, 54a
Teaching Aids at Low Cost: 67
The Mansell Collection, London: 7, 8, 9, 11, 12, 13,
15, 58
Dr M J G Thomas: 18, 32b, 40a
Topham Picture Library: 3, 76
Wellcome Institute Library, London: 48, 71
**Audio Visual Dept, Western Ophthalmic Hospital,
London:** 21
World Health Organisation: 16, 79, 80, 82

Figures 29, 33, and 36 were redrawn from "Atlas of
Medical Helminthology and Protozoology", Jeffrey
and Leach with permission from Churchill Livingstone.

Contents

Preface

It is easy to get complacent about infection. The British Medical Association thinks that it would be very unwise to do so.

We live in a world of infection. To keep us free from infectious disease takes ceaseless vigilance. As patients sit snuffling in their waiting rooms, doctors are only too aware that upper respiratory disorders (to name only one group of infectious disease) are responsible for countless hours of lost work, and thus of production and of money – not to mention yet more countless hours of low-grade misery at home. As the doctor examines a patient for an unexplained fever, he must now take account of the possibility of recent travel or immigration, and thus the carriage of a disease which although rare in the richer parts of the world is all too common to medical practitioners in less favoured nations.

At the supermarket, the contented shopper chooses a toilet cleanser to destroy '99% of all household germs' (for whatever good that would do), and moves on to the chicken counter little knowing that the odds are that many of the fowls on display are riddled with salmonella bacteria, one of the commonest causes of food poisoning. At home, almost everyone may now assume that the water from kitchen taps is safe to drink, but be unaware of the stringent efforts needed to keep it that way, or of the difficulty in separating sewage from it. Eating at a restaurant in town, the family has no idea whether or not minute scraps of excreta have unwittingly been transferred to the plates of food by the smiling waiter.

Several widespread assumptions are groundless. For instance, high-tech homes and kitchens cannot guarantee safety. Gleaming refrigerators cannot ensure that food will stay free from contamination and toxins, and the belief that foodstuffs are always hygienically packaged and handled before purchase may be unwarranted. And, if by some misfortune a virulent bug does cause infectious disease, it is not always true that a suitable antibiotic will be available to kill it.

With present efforts to combat infection apparently successful, it may well be believed that there is very little need to worry about infection at all. Over the past twenty years 'new' diseases have emerged, among them legionellosis and Lassa fever. However, others will no doubt follow as scientific research isolates organisms and uncovers their association with clinical disease. Many may well be found to be of infectious origin. Although the risk of serious infectious disease is now truly very low in Britain, the reader will find many examples in this book of how such carefree assumptions may be groundless.

Constant attention to the details of infection control, therefore, is needed at community level and personal level alike. To highlight the need for such vigilance is the purpose of this book.

Particular attention has been paid to infectious diseases which are of special interest to people in Britain. But micro-organisms are not particularly impressed by the fact that Britain is an island, and therefore the control of infectious disease has been placed in a global context. In the less fortunate and poorer parts of the world, serious infectious diseases are still rife and are often the biggest killers of all, sparing neither young nor old. Boundaries between the developing nations and the developed world are insubstantial at best, which represents a double risk: that travellers can pick up strange infections when away from home, and that they may export their own domestic diseases to their destinations abroad. No longer can it be assumed that distance – or the English Channel – means isolation. An infectious disease which creeps over such insubstantial boundaries may find a population quite unprepared for its attack, and very vulnerable to it. The first world is openly exposed to the infections of the third.

The intention of this book is to cover a wide range of matters related to 'infection control', from the washing of hands to the worldwide eradication of smallpox. Emphasis has been placed on the process of infection and its control rather than on the study of individual infections, but some diseases are either so important or so intrinsically interesting that special attention has been given to them, more, perhaps, than their frequency in Britain would seem to justify. Citizens of other parts of the world do not share in this good fortune, and still have to battle the diseases which we have eradicated from our shores.

Many examples of notable diseases have been used, too, to show how knowledge of infection control has steadily developed over the years. The history of infection control is a human story, full of the names of Nobel Laureates and of others who have fallen as martyrs to the diseases they were studying.

This volume is not intended as a textbook of public health, microbiology or sanitary science, and will replace no such publications. Diagnosis and treatment are also matters for detailed and specialised texts. The intention has been to place the subject of infection control in the context of mankind's great struggle with deprivation and disease, taking into account the human relationship with the natural world and all its creatures, microscopic organisms included.

It should therefore be of interest to all who are concerned with the world around them, and with how human beings interact with its natural elements. It should be of practical use to non-medical people whose duties and interests embrace management of the environment as a means to infection control; these could include, for example, sanitary engineers and executive or managerial personnel in the food industry. And, of course, apart from members of the medical profession and medical students, it should have particular appeal to science students and to nurses and members of associated health professions.

Infectious disease too often results from failure to apply what we know. Infection control requires involvement. Involvement needs interest, and it is interest in this engrossing topic which we have tried to arouse in this book.

This volume was prepared under the auspices of the Board of Science and Education of the British Medical Association. The members of the Board during its preparation were as follows:

Sir Douglas Black – Chairman (to July 1988)
Sir Christopher Booth – Chairman (from July 1988)
Professor J P Payne – Deputy Chairman
Dr G Adams
Dr A Carney
Dr J M Cundy
Dr M Goodman
Dr J R W Hangartner (from July 1988)
Dr M F Hudson (from July 1988)
Major General J M Matheson
Dr G M Mitchell
Dr V Moens
Professor J P Quilliam
Dr M J G Thomas

A Steering Group with the following membership assisted in the preparation of the report:

Dr W M Dixon
Dr L F Fisher
Dr C L Smith
Dr M J G Thomas

Introduction

The control of infection is a fascinating subject. The very course of the history of mankind has been changed by great epidemic diseases of the past, which swept across continents and were brought under human control in recent years only. Control of such mighty scourges was the daunting challenge of the past; the less dramatic but equally important challenge of the present is to sustain our success in keeping down the rate of serious infectious disease to its presently low level. The battle against severe infectious disease has not been lightly won, and it continues unabated in the developing world. It is no easy matter to maintain control over the micro-organisms whose capacity for adaptation to adversity is so much greater than ours.

Infection control is necessary even in the most highly developed countries because:

- free movement and communications make the spread of infection across national borders an ever-present possibility, and serious infectious disease is still the major cause of death in the developing countries;

- infectious respiratory disease remains uncontrolled and is a continuing burden on public and personal resources;

- food and water are commonly far from free from injurious micro-organisms, and what are generally regarded as minor illnesses such as food poisoning are increasing;

- bacteria are becoming increasingly resistant to antibiotics;

- there are very few drugs available for the treatment of diseases caused by viruses; and

- viruses probably cause more diseases than we now realise.

This book describes how infectious disease is controlled in both developed and developing nations, because regions of the world cannot be considered in isolation where infection is concerned, and because in many ways the third world now faces the same problems of control that the developed world successfully overcame not so long ago.

The key to the control of an infectious disease is understanding how it is spread, and due emphasis has been placed on this fact in structuring the book. Every infection must have been transmitted from someone or somewhere, and it follows that to stop transmission is to stop the disease. This has been successfully done for many diseases in many regions – after centuries as a killer, the transmission of yellow fever in Central America was stopped in a matter of months, following discovery of the way it was spread – and in one instance, smallpox, transmission has been stopped all over the world. This awful disease has been rendered extinct.

The different kinds of micro-organisms and the diseases they cause are described, the processes in the body which arise to combat them, the way they spread and persist in the community, and the special technique man has developed to fight infectious disease. We all have considerable scope in the way we organise our lives and make day-to-day decisions on our activities and behaviour, in order to reduce to a minimum the risk of both contracting and passing on infection.

In Chapter 1, infectious disease has been set in an ecological context. Man and microbes share this world, and have done so for millions of years. The microbes were here first, and have a much greater capacity than man for adapting and changing in response to environmental circumstances. What man does is to change the environment to suit himself. In so doing, he changes his relationship with the microbes, sometimes increasing the risk that they may cause him disease, and sometimes decreasing it. When disease-causing micro-organisms are newly introduced into man's environment the effect can be devastating, with the fatal impact of smallpox in the new Spanish colonies, measles in the Pacific islands and cholera in Europe all being dramatic examples.

The dawning of a new science, that of bacteriology, is described in Chapter 2. In early times no-one had the faintest idea of what was causing infectious disease, yet some of the worst epidemics were brought under control by determined men whose broader aim was to improve the dreadful living conditions of the Middle Ages and the years that followed. They fomented the sanitary revolution, and the reason for their success was shown later by the research of workers such as Pasteur, whose work was of such fundamental importance to our understanding of the nature of microscopic life that their names literally became part of the language. The paths outlined by these pioneers

were later to be followed by whole nations, latterly united in the great spirit of international cooperation embodied in the World Health Organisation.

The new understanding brought about by the work of such men led to an amazing change in the pattern of disease in many parts of the world, with the degenerative changes of old age, and accidents among the young, replacing infection as the great causes of premature death. These changes are outlined in Chapter 3. The pattern of infection has itself been changed, with the emergence of infectious diseases newly recognised as threats: legionellosis, AIDS, hepatitis B, Lassa fever and many others. The microbes themselves, and many of the diseases they cause, are the subject of Chapter 4. With many of the bacteria – the staphylococci, the streptococci – we are in general quite familiar. But with others, such as the chlamydiae, we are having to come to terms very quickly, because it seems that they are behind many diseases we did not know the causes of before.

Viruses, too, are almost certainly causing more illness than we now recognise or can currently demonstrate, as well as being responsible for the familiar respiratory ailments which make life such a misery for so many so often. The protozoa cause illness and death among millions of people in the warmer countries of the world, including perhaps the most widespread and important disease man has ever had to tackle, malaria. This was once a common cause of death in Britain, and is still the commonest protozoal disease to be imported.

Colonisation by micro-organisms does not always lead to infectious disease. Bacterial invasion does not inevitably make us sick. Man swarms with micro-organisms which do him no harm. Why some make him ill, and how the human body responds to microbial invasion, are the subjects of Chapter 5. Many aspects of infection control are aimed at modifying the interaction between man and microbes, and bolstering the body's defences against the potentially injurious invaders.

Chapter 6 covers the spread of disease, the key to control. Spread can be in many ways: by way of food and drink, in the air, by direct contact, and through the intermediary action of animals and insects. In this chapter we outline many examples of infectious disease in the context of the way each one is spread; naturally, control of a disease spread by sexual contact will be a fundamentally different matter from control of one which is spread by the bite of a mosquito.

This theme is continued in Chapter 7, where specific examples of control measures are examined including such disparate activities as the purification of sewage and the preparation of food in the home. The control of diseases spread by insects is a matter of particular importance to the tropical world, and requires understanding and control of the insects themselves.

There are several categories of control which cover the whole field of infection. Immunisation is one, a measure which has had startling success in decimating the incidence of some of the most feared illnesses of all, such as poliomyelitis and diphtheria. Disinfection and sterilisation have been essential to safe and clean surgery, and the development and use of antibiotics have been vital contributors to control activities. These are all, in their way, technical fields; but the other subjects covered in Chapter 8 are of personal importance to all people, technical, medical or otherwise. These are personal hygiene and the particular problems faced by travellers in places where standards of hygiene and medical care may not be as high as those to which we are accustomed in Britain, North America or Australasia.

In the final chapter we review some great efforts by the international community to control infectious disease at the global level, taking particular account of the spectacular success of the World Health Organisation together with many individual nations in ridding the world of smallpox. Such massive efforts at infection control have lessons at regional, local and personal levels, and those lessons are drawn on at the close of the book.

Appendix A consists of an alphabetical list of sources of further information on the control of infection, and on infectious disease generally. Many are regarded as standard medical texts (Christie, for example) but others are aimed at more general reading (Dawood, for instance, and Howe). In Appendix B some of the more important micro-organisms are listed for quick reference, including a brief note on their most common sources, the diseases they cause, and therapeutic agents typically used to treat them.

Just because measures to control infection have been so successful in countries such as Britain, there is a great temptation to ease up on them. This would be a great mistake. History has shown how terrible the effect on mankind the spread of infection can be, and it would be foolish in the extreme to ignore the lessons of history. Complacency is the kiss of death to infection control.

Infection and Ecology

THE STRUGGLE FOR HEALTH

The paradox is this. We daily face the threat of infectious disease, and serious pathogens are not far away. Yet, as figures demonstrate, the infections that do make us ill are mostly minor ones. Why, then, the fuss?

It is true, certainly, that man no longer faces the great epidemic diseases of the past, dreams of which can mentally portray giant armies of virulent bacteria marching off to war, antigens glowing, a battle to the death in the offing. Such images do die very hard. Just consider, for example, the shock and horror generated by reports of a single case of typhoid or – worse, perhaps – leprosy, especially if described in suitably lurid terms. It is implied that such diseases are simply lying in wait, ready to leap out on us once again. This is, of course, utter nonsense. The situation is that most bacteria and most human beings live pretty happily together in peace, and not in a state of continual conflict. Sometimes, infection leads to illness. Often, it does not.

The central theme of this book is that man and the microbes have reached a state of accommodation, in precarious balance. In Britain and the developed world, the balance is in man's favour. In poor and hungry nations, the scales are tipped the other way. In order to *keep* things in our favour, and to try to improve things in the developing world, it is essential that we watch the balance and deliberately weight the scales if possible. That process is what we mean by 'control'. If serious infectious disease were common, there would be no need to argue the need for control. But when such disease is rare, as a result of past successes, it is easy to forget that control remains as important as ever.

The World Health Organisation (WHO), in the glow of optimism surrounding the writing of its constitution, defined health as 'a state of complete physical, mental and social well-being, and not merely the absence of disease or infirmity'. Dictionary definitions of health also tend to the absolute. But health is not an absolute. Certainly, the achievement of 'complete' well-being is a bold and desirable objective, but a more practical expression of the idea of health is that it represents a state of being which allows effective (and some might add happy) functioning within a given environment, reasonably free of pain, disability or limitation of action. The present aim of the WHO is to make possible the attainment by all citizens of the world by the year 2000 of a level of health that will permit them to lead a socially and economically productive life.

The 'healthy' body is in a position to meet potentially threatening changes in the external environment swiftly and efficiently. To do that, the body's own internal environment needs to be in a state of contented equilibrium, because when that equilibrium breaks down, illness is likely. 'Homeostasis', from Greek words meaning literally 'staying the same', is a term which has been used to describe the harmonious state which allows the body to cope with changes in the external environment. A disturbance of homeostasis can allow infectious invaders in.

Illness therefore represents a pattern of response by the individual body to harmful forces in the environment, outside him, on him, and within him. A wide variety of parasites – a term which we use here in its biological sense to embrace all micro-organisms, including bacteria – exist in man's environment, and they can therefore get caught up in the sort of environmental change which represents a threat to the individual and his health. For each case of illness, however, they are far from being the only 'cause'.

Even those bacteria which are capable of causing disease may only do so in a semi-accidental manner, being under normal circumstances residents of some part of the human body and known as 'commensals'. Just as a forest is carpeted with flora, so it is that our body is densely colonised by bacterial 'flora'. Most become *pathogenic* – that is, produce disease – only under the most unusual circumstances. Thus, the notion that the only good germ is a dead germ is absurd, because the vast majority of micro-organisms have nothing to do with diseases of man. Indeed, many of the microbes with which we are living in a balanced and contented relationship are actually protecting us from infectious disease. If we kill them off, for example through the injudicious use of antibiotic drugs, only too often what can occur is an illness caused by new and opportunistic invaders who have marched into an empty field, and who are likely to be resistant to the drugs which have seen off their predecessors.

Pathological organisms frequently colonise the body – 'the host' – but this rarely results in disease. Infection is the invasion of the host by pathogenic organisms under environmental circumstances which allow them to do harm. But even then, colonisation does not necessarily result in damage, and most infections do not result in disease.

When outright infectious disease does occur, it represents one of the host's reactions to the invading pathogen, and the actual course of the illness will be affected by characteristics of both the host and the invader. These will be examined in more detail later in this book. But, briefly, the most important attributes of the invading organism are:

- *pathogenicity*, which is its actual ability to produce disease;
- *infectivity*, its ability to spread from person to person;
- *invasiveness*, its ability to spread within the host;
- *virulence*, which affects the severity of the illness; and
- *the number* of invaders involved in the attack.

Looking to the host, among the most important determinants of any resulting disease will be age, sex, and hormonal and genetic factors. These will interact with the individual's immune status, and all add up to what is generally known as 'resistance'.

Man has had some spectacular successes in controlling infectious disease. In the space of a few decades we have seen the absolute eradication of one infectious disease, smallpox; the virtual elimination (particularly in the developed world) of many other diseases, such as diphtheria and poliomyelitis, which were truly terrifying killers; the bringing of other scourges under strict regional control; and the invention of medicines which seem to promise prevention or cure for most of the infectious illnesses that remain. The success of steps which were taken in the early days must have seemed miraculous. And when people realised that invisibly tiny organisms were at the root of it all, it was little wonder that they thought: 'At last! Medicine is coming really to understand diseases, so that we can identify the one cause for each, and identify the unique cure for it'.

Alas, the world is not as simple as that. One of the great pioneers in infection control, René Dubos, wrote in *The Mirage of Health*:

'The very process of living is a continual interplay between the individual and his environment, often taking the form of a struggle resulting in injury or disease.'

It is clear, therefore, that not even diseases 'caused' by microbes result from microbes alone. Inter-related factors struggle for supremacy, knotted together in a complex web, and ill health is a consequence of several of those factors acting together. Four billion people harbour potentially pathogenic micro-organisms, but do not develop any disease. A child in Kensington ingests some bacteria. It stays off school for the day. A child in Ethiopia ingests the same. But it sickens and dies.

PEOPLE AND PARASITES: THE UNEASY BALANCE

Thus, man shares this world with bacteria and many other potentially damaging micro-organisms, and must work out a relationship with them. In fact, of course, they were here some thousands of million years before man, and the acceptable partnership we have with them is a feature of the inter-acting system composed of living organisms which is called the ecosystem.

After bacteria were first identified, biologists and others interested in the study of mankind concentrated on them as objects in their own right, and on their intrinsic characteristics. This concentration was initially at the expense of concern with

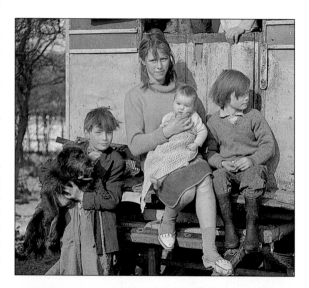

Figure 1 Our suscepti-bility to invading micro-organisms varies greatly according to who we are and how we live.

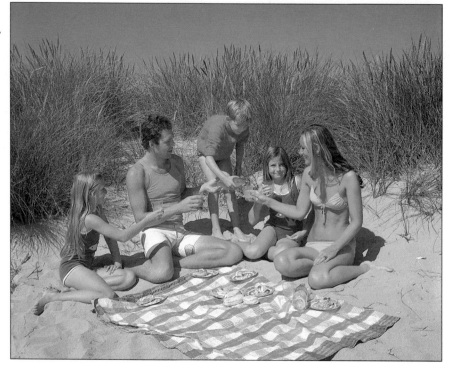

the way they fit into the whole scheme of things, how they share man's environment and how the balance swings between infection and disease.

The density of a population is one of the critical factors in determining the stability of a balanced relationship, and consequently the chances of survival of its members. This is true whether we are talking about micro-organisms, lower animals, or human beings. A dense population is open to attack by those that will themselves succeed by preying upon it. Take a simple example. Chickens are subject to a parasitic infection. They excrete the parasites in their faeces, and then pick them up when faeces contaminate their food. Suppose there are ten chickens in a big yard, and one of them excretes the parasite. There is a chance then that one of the other nine will pick up the parasite, but there's plenty of ground to peck over, transmission through the flock is likely to be slow, and the chickens are as a group unlikely to suffer greatly. On the other hand, suppose that the population in the same yard is increased to 500 chickens. There is then 50 times the risk that another chicken will pick up the parasite – and so on, with the parasite spreading like lightning through the flock and reinfection making the resulting sickness worse.

Again in the real world, something of the same sort occurs when plagues of little animals like mice break out, as quite often happens in rural Australia. When that happens, the nightly television news is full of alarming pictures of tumbling hordes of mice, gazed upon by happy cats and despairing farmers, who cannot see any end to the infestation as numbers escalate daily.

But one day a mouse or two is seen dead, infected by a micro-organism which is strange to it. Then others die in their millions as the infection sweeps through the susceptible horde, and the mouse population recedes to the number at which it was originally in equilibrium with its environment.

There have been similar, though less dramatic

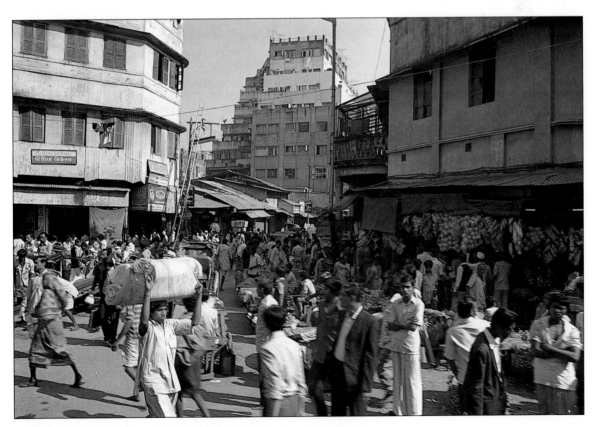

Figure 2 Crowded street, Calcutta. The density of a population affects the ease and speed of transmission of infection.

ups and downs, in the growth of the number of the human race. In rural areas, food is adequate, numbers grow, and sooner or later groups of people drift towards the centres of population. The history of the ancient world is full of stories of mass migrations to what were at first the original city states, but which later evolved into the great urban conglomerates with which we are now so familiar. But the closely packed urban environment of the early days allowed infectious disease to flourish, and many pathogenic parasites succeeded at man's expense, so providing a check on the rise of his burgeoning population until again a new balance was reached. As is seen so sadly in the famine-struck areas of the world today, population control through the holocaust of mass starvation is a horrible course of events; however, infections caused by the organisms which flourish in such conditions were for centuries the main way in which human populations were stabilised. This phenomenon was first recognised by Malthus (1766–1834), who observed that the populations in these urban communities outgrew their food supplies. Widespread malnutrition followed, the people then becoming susceptible to infection. He saw this as nature's way of controlling over-population; hence the term Malthusian checks. Evidence of such Malthusian checks can be found in the reports of the great plagues: the Black Death for example, and in the outbreaks of cholera in nineteenth century cities (Soho in London for example in 1854).

When a parasite is newly introduced into a human population which has not been exposed to it before – as in the case of the Australian mice – the effects can be disastrous. This was seen throughout the Pacific Ocean during the eighteenth century, as western man extended his explorations and activities there. As one example, Captain Cook's crews laid a trail of sexually transmitted diseases through the entire South Seas, to the great cost of their friendly people. As another, a Fiji chief returning from a trip to England brought with him the measles virus, which exploded throughout the Fiji archipelago and resulted in the death of some one-fifth of the whole population. Once established in a new relationship, however, the measles virus and man in Fiji settled into equilibrium. Since that awful epidemic, the incidence of the disease has been about the same as anywhere else, including, for example, the British Isles from which it came. An epidemic loses all its steam when

there are no longer enough people susceptible to infection by the available pathogens.

The ecological balance between man and the parasites which make their living on him is a special one and sometimes rather uneasy, because there are two groups of organisms involved. The first group can be categorised as those that come from the outside, and are termed 'exogenous'. Among these are the viruses of measles and small-pox. They are not normally found around man-kind to any great extent, and there has been no opportunity to evolve a working relationship. When man encounters such parasites, battle is almost inevitable.

On the other hand, there are those many para-sitic micro-organisms with which man lives quite normally and perfectly happily, the 'endogenous' variety. They include, for example, the billions upon billions of the bacteria which live in his intes-tines, without some of which he could not even digest his food. Some of these can occasionally cause illness – but considering the number that are there all the time, somewhere between a thousand million and a million million, they do so surpris-ingly rarely. Just why everyone is not ill all the time is one of the things that we set out to explain in this book. But to return to the point: man has reached a stable and amicable working relationship with the endogenous group of parasites. Of course, this is an oversimplification – there are many organisms which could be fitted into either group – but the underlying difference in relation-ship is there, and it has important implications for the control of infectious disease.

Infectious disease, it follows from the above dis-cussion, is but a special example of the interaction between man and parasites: when illness strikes, it represents a state of conflict. When the host and the parasite are in a balanced relationship, disease is unusual and death very rare; what is normal is infection which is 'unapparent', or 'subclinical'. In simple terms, we build up resistance to these familiar microbes.

Conflict is more likely when the environment is changing, and equilibrium more likely when the environment stays constant. But a characteristic of modern man is that he keeps changing the envi-ronment. Accordingly, conflict with and attack by parasites is in principle likely, and likely to result in infectious disease, unless countervailing factors are introduced in order to restore the balance. And these, of course, will include the control measures which this book sets out to describe.

Although man can and does change his environment rather easily and rather quickly, he cannot change himself. Over a period of thousands of years, man has retained basically the same genetic make-up. That is assuredly not the case for the microbes. They can reproduce so fast that their inherited characteristics can change very rapidly too – a generation of E. coli bacteria flashes by in about 20 minutes, compared to around 30 years in the case of humans. It follows that diseases which are prevalent throughout a human population – endemic – are very hard to eliminate because the parasites change in subtle ways, weighting the environmental balance in their favour. The best example of this is the influenza virus.

Practically everything is a host or a parasite to something else. In the famous words of Jonathan Swift:

> 'So, naturalists observe, a flea
> Hath smaller fleas that on him prey;
> And these have smaller fleas to bite 'em,
> And so proceed *ad infinitum*.'

A balanced relationship is usually a successful one, and as such, balances may have existed for many generations. Microbes have been around a lot longer than man on this world, and vigorous attempts to see them all dead and gone will do no good, and could well do him harm. However, some exogenous pathogens do have terrible effects on human beings uniquely, and it may indeed be possible, without disturbing the ecological balance of the world, to eradicate them completely. Diseases caused by such microbes include smallpox and malaria, and there are other diseases, such as rabies, which have indeed been completely eliminated in particular parts of the world with no environmental ill effects.

THE ENVIRONMENTAL BATTLEFIELD

So far, we have concentrated on the relationship of the host, man, with the parasite – the 'agent' – that infects him and, sometimes, causes infectious disease. Man and the agent of illness are two elements of a triad which has become a classic part of epidemiology (which is the study of diseases throughout whole communities rather than in individuals.

The environment is the third element of that triad. All of the diseases and disorders which trouble mankind can be assessed with the host/agent/environment triad forming the conceptual base. Even road accidents, and the terrible toll of death and injury that they wreak, can be considered in this context; man is the road user, mechanical energy is the agent of injury, and these two components are interacting in the environment of the third, the roadway. This analogy even extends to regarding the road vehicle as the 'vector' which carries the agent of injury, just as the mosquito vector carries the malaria parasite to the victim. Such a concept revolutionised approaches to the reduction of traffic injury, because it highlighted the intimate interaction of the three elements and made it easy to promote the idea that if the environment were to be changed, then that could improve safety as much as or more than efforts to change human behaviour.

Infectious disease is as much a phenomenon with multiple causes as is traffic injury. For example, while the typhoid bacillus is the necessary agent for causing the disease, outbreaks are determined not only by the presence of the bacillus but also by the cleanliness of water supplies, how sewage is disposed of and so on. And, of course, it was those who concentrated on the environment in attempting to control infection who first showed the way to reduction in human losses from infectious disease. When we examine the history of infectious disease control in the next chapter, we will see in much greater detail how the environment was successfully manipulated, and in later chapters we review specific measures appropriate to the modern day. For the moment, however, we simply seek to establish some principles.

Man's essential being – his genetic make-up – changes with incredible slowness as the generations pass, as we have already noted. Man's behaviour can be changed, but only with great difficulty, because behaviour is so intimately related to culture, upbringing and well-established traits. For everyone to boil all tap water at home would certainly ease the load of administrators who are seeking to eliminate water-borne infections – but it would be a foolish administrator who would rely on exhortation and education about boiling water rather than on purifying the water at its source.

Man's capacity for changing the environment gives him his capacity to control it, and thus to

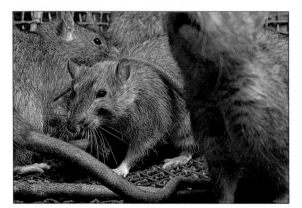

Figure 3   When the numbers in a population grow too fast, and expand into plague proportions, they become susceptible to infectious diseases. A number of them will die, thus restoring equilibrium with the environment.

control the incidence of infectious disease. In modern times, at least, man in essence creates his own environment. It is therefore well within his capacity to adapt it to his advantage.

Parasites, at the same time, are seeking the most desirable environment for themselves. In one which favours them, they will multiply their numbers up to a state of equilibrium, and the risk of infectious disease is thereby higher than if their numbers were limited to a lower level by an environment which is unfavourable for them. In most instances, the conditions which favour micro-organisms are those which do not favour man, and *vice versa*. So, for all sorts of reasons, it makes sense for man to tackle those parts of the environment he is able to, with a view not only to making things pleasant for himself, but also to making things highly unpleasant for those creatures that would do him harm if they could.

Of course, that is just what man has been trying to do over the years. But many of the environmental changes he has deliberately brought about have favoured micro-organisms at his own expense. As people pack into urban communities, crowding increases the chance of transmitting infection borne on droplets in the air. It puts strain on sanitary engineering. It makes the supply of clean water and food increasingly difficult. Now that the relationship of all such factors to the risk of infectious disease is understood, we can be on wary lookout, and try to keep up with such environmental changes, so that they are not swamped by pressures of population. But in many parts of the

third world today it simply may not be possible to force environmental change fast enough to keep up with the threat of infectious disease, even though the mechanisms of spread are perfectly well known, at least to health administrators. Such places are now roughly in the situation seen in earlier times in the now developed world, when people began migrating into the cities and placing impossible strains on public services.

Not that what we would now call the public service infrastructure was there in those early days, even in the biggest cities. When people thought disease was spread by smell and vapours, rather than by flies and water, there was little perceived need for attention to sanitary measures. Administrators could blame the people for the conditions – the lower classes for their filthy way of life – so pressures for environmental change were light or non-existent.

Fortunately, however, some enlightened individuals set out vigorously to combat the squalor. That they played a large role in defeating infectious disease was partly a lucky by-product of their endeavours, but it happened nevertheless. The names of some of these men will appear later in these pages. They were the pioneers who helped to

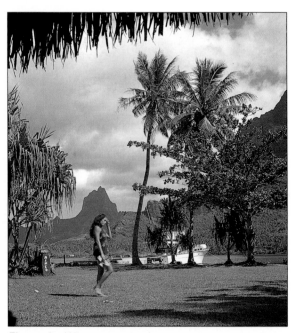

Figure 4   When organisms are newly introduced into an environment, the people have no resistance to them and epidemic disease is likely.

make serious infectious disease a rarity in the cities of the developed world today

An ironical sidelight on the importance of the environment in determining how we live and die is to be discerned in the new pattern of disease in cities of the modern western world. The major maladies now are the non-infectious ones: the heart problems, the accidental injuries, and the degenerative and cancerous conditions initiated by our life style, and developing to the full during the long life now allowed us by our freedom from serious infection.

The clean-up of the cities happened to coincide with the emergence of two scientific disciplines, those of epidemiology and bacteriology. Scientists in the first group were able to identify what was happening in the environment, and make adaptations to change things for the better. Snow's removal of the handle of the Broad Street pump (described in the next chapter) is perhaps the simplest and best-known example of such an action. The actual mechanisms underlying the changes which made things better were unknown. But then came the bacteriologists, to show how it was that microscopic organisms were the essential causes of infectious disease. This was such an illuminating observation that it was thought, erroneously, that microbes were the cause of infectious disease – and it took some sad experiments to show that control of just the microbes was only one

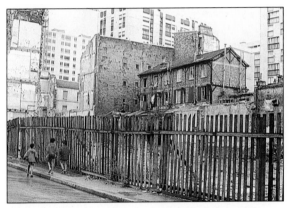

Figure 6   Poor housing and overcrowding add to the risk of infection by easing the transmission of pathogenic organisms and lowering the general level of health.

small step towards dealing with the problem as a whole.

The key elements for creating an environment which makes things good for man and bad for pathogenic microbes are, it may seem to us now, perfectly obvious. They include:

- an adequate supply of water which is clean and free from bacteria, water which man can safely drink, swim in and use for washing himself and his clothes;

- the availability of food which is supplied free of pathogenic bacteria and other parasites; and

- the disposal of sewage, refuse and industrial waste in such a manner that bacteria proliferate in a controlled manner such that the sites of disposal cannot become breeding grounds for vectors of infectious disease such as rats and flies.

But to state such things is not to have them happen. A reliable supply of pure water is increasingly hard to ensure, and even in many developed countries the residents prefer to rely on bottles of water bought from the local supermarket (although the purity of bottled water is not yet a matter for standardisation and regulatory control). Run-off from agricultural areas can contaminate water supplies with animal manure and chemical fertilisers. The problem of refuse disposal in large cities has reached such proportions that available landfill area is almost exhausted, and man may

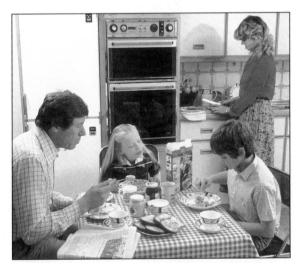

Figure 5   The modern household has a plentiful supply of clean water, refrigerated food and adequate waste disposal systems; all the necessary elements of a world free from infectious disease.

turn for resolution of his disposal problems to other parts of his environment, such as the sea, thus imposing new strains on the ecosystem. The supply of mass-processed food has in many ways made the assurance of its quality harder – the contamination of chickens with Salmonella is one example – and the popularity of eating out these days has meant that an increasing number of food handlers are inexperienced and badly trained.

Housing is similarly a public health responsibility, because cramped, crowded and poorly ventilated dwellings suit the bacteria more than man, and allow them to reach equilibrium at numbers which pose a threat. Light and airy surroundings at work and at home make infectious disease less likely, whereas those who have no home at all face a disproportionate risk of infection. However, in our efforts to improve matters and clean up the environment, we may have taken some ill-advised turnings. Rat-infested, poorly-ventilated terraced slums were with all good intentions torn down; but many people were then compelled to live in blocks of flats which towered over their surroundings, and the very isolation which was lowering the risk of infectious disease went on to cause some of the 'new' non-infectious disorders of poorly stress-adapted modern man.

But, again, man has the capacity to change things, and there are no steps which cannot be retraced. Man has to make sure that he does not regress to the situation he was in before, remembering also that at times of social upheaval – and at all times in some places – environmental measures may be easily disrupted. The history of the control of the great diseases is an absorbing one, and it is to that story which we now turn. But we should never forget, as we do so, that what is past history for us is present day for many others in the world.

2

The Coming
of a Science

EARLY DAYS

The control of infectious disease has an inspiring history. Even more than most such stories in medicine, it on the one hand serves to deepen our appreciation of the heroic efforts of the past and, on the other, helps us to learn from past failures and make them less likely in the future. It is a history which still unfolds; while in the developed world man wrestles with the new complexities of civilisation and the associated diseases which are now the main killers, in other parts of the globe the battle is still with the infections and the epidemics with which our predecessors fought in centuries long gone.

Primitive man worshipped the sun, the moon, the stars, and many other features of the natural world around him. Many people in the world still do. The common factor is animism, the belief that the world abounds with invisible spirits that determine everything that happens. These spirits may be much feared, and are believed sometimes to enter our world in animate form. Among the hill tribes of Thailand, twin babies are both killed after birth because one of them is assumed to be a spirit come into being: but which one, it is impossible to

know, and the spirit cannot be allowed to survive in human form.

In Anglo-Saxon England, spirits were believed to emerge in the form of clouds or gaseous vapours from marshes, and pestilence (a term originally used to refer to any epidemic disease) stalked the land in finite form in the guise of a loathly monster', whose touch would bring inevitable death.

For centuries the approaches to, and treatment of, disease were but part of the system by which angry spirits and gods were appeased. The influential personality assigned to the treatment and prevention of disease in any one community would be the one who would also be required to assure good crops and the bringing of rain. Disease was but one of the works of an evil spirit, and treatment consisted of driving it out by what is now called magic but which seemed then – given acceptance of the premise of cause – an entirely rational approach. The prevention and treatment of disease through the apparently analytical use of remedies based on erroneous theories of causation continued even in the western world until very close to the present day.

Pictorial writing from thousands of years before Christ has shown that Babylonian physicians regarded disease as the work of demons, and clay tablets of the time describe the formulation of medicines to be used to support incantations in the driving out of sickness. The early Egyptian civilisation was another that left good records, and they similarly reveal the belief of citizens of the Nile Valley of some 3000 to 1000 BC that angry gods would punish the people with plagues and illness; an idea which, in the case of sexually transmitted diseases, still has plenty of running in it. In relation to prevention, the Egyptians of that era had already identified the benefits of a sound diet and good personal hygiene, and they were perhaps the first to document their belief that the vapours from decomposing flesh would cause disease: this was, basically, the theory of miasma, which prevailed in Britain until only a century or so ago.

Away to the east, but also some thousands of years ago, it was probably in India that inoculation by the fluid from the vesicles of smallpox was first used to prevent the disease. The Chinese also knew of this procedure, and another technique that employed acupuncture to promote balance between competing forces in the body, a concept akin to that of homeostasis.

Among the Semitic peoples the idea that sin was the root cause of disease is seen fully developed in the writings of the Old Testament, which contains scores of references to the use by the Lord of plagues to punish the unrighteous; and forgiveness of sin, in the New Testament, is associated with the curing of disease. The Jewish people originated many of the principles of public hygiene, and their religious food laws must have spared them much of the illness which was rife among their contemporaries.

The emergence of the great civilisation of ancient Greece, and the philosophical and scientific revolution it brought, was based in part on the studies and writings of the Egyptian people, whom the Greeks had been visiting for hundreds of years. The close scientific association of these two civilisations was to continue. But it was uniquely the Greeks who introduced a truly revolutionary concept, one which became a turning point in human thought: that the world, and indeed the universe, was part of a system which could be explained on the basis of discoverable laws and measurable parameters. If diseases and other natural phenomena were the result of supernatural influences, then clearly there was nothing that man could do about them; but if man was in charge of

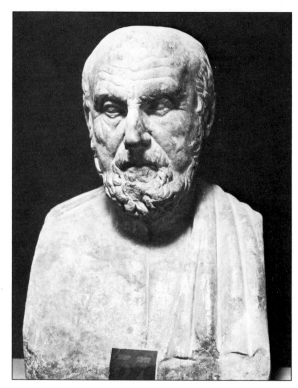

Figure 7 Hippocrates, who laid the scientific foundations of medicine.

his destiny, then in principle there was nothing he could not do.

Hippocrates, who lived from 460 to 370 BC, has been called the father of medicine, and as well as so famously expressing its ethical ideals he gave medicine its scientific spirit. He and the people who worked with him had little or no knowledge of anatomy or physiology, but they obtained their results by combining application of their own logic and common sense with faith in the patient's natural powers of recovery. Among other insights, the Hippocratic school recognised the difference between endemic and epidemic disease, and identified the influence of climate and weather on illness.

It was the biologist Aristotle, born 14 years before the death of Hippocrates, who founded the natural sciences, and his writings were to provide intellectual stimulus to European scientists for the next 2000 years. Soon after his death the Egyptian connection was confirmed by the building of a medical school at Alexandria, staffed by Greek physicians. The last of the great Greek physicians of the period was Galen, who in fact worked most

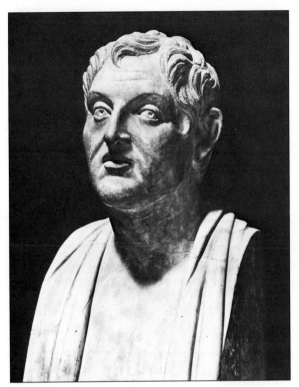

Figure 8 Aristotle, the founder of the natural sciences.

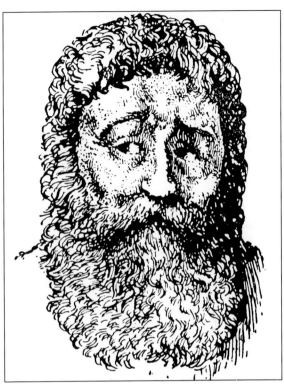

Figure 9 Galen, the last of the great Greek physicians of the ancient world.

of his life (131–201 AD) in Egypt and in Rome. A voluminous writer, he was so influential that his concepts were regarded as the final authority until well into the eighteenth century. But they were vague, and based on ideas of spirits and humours. Galen shied away from facts which could be demonstrated empirically, a concept which had been promoted by Hippocrates, and substituted theorisation for observation and deduction. Perhaps this was why Galen was so popular with some medical scientists for so long. Having to prove things can be very difficult when it comes to improvements in health. As put neatly by Hilaire Belloc:

'Oh! Let us never, never doubt
What nobody is sure about!'

The approach of the Roman civilisation to medical problems was based on the thinking of the Greeks, but translated into practical form. Public health was their strong point. They planned their towns from scratch, and municipal life was a feature of Roman civilisation; in Britain alone they built about 50 new cities in the south of the country. Their streets were wide and well-paved, their buildings solid and built of stone and bricks. The houses of the more prosperous were often heated by underfloor chambers, and public bath-houses became popular meeting places. Throughout their empire they piped in running water: the aqueducts of Rome, which brought water from up the River Tiber and from wells, delivered at their peak over 200 million gallons a day. At points along the aqueducts settling tanks were constructed in order to allow solid particles to settle out, and because of its purity, this water was reserved for drinking. Many Roman cities had sewerage systems for the disposal of waste, and some latrines – such as the ones in Hadrian's Wall – were flushed by running water.

In the Middle Ages, after the collapse of Rome, people of the west turned to the church as the fount of wisdom, and theories of the supernatural origin of disease once again held sway. Scientific method was not opposed, it was simply viewed as irrelevant. For almost eight centuries it was once again held that almost all disease was the result of the actions of demonic spirits, and a popular counter-measure of the time was the burning of those deemed to be witches. In the east, however, schools and libraries flourished and physicians continued to build a scientific base, and as Islam swept west in the seventh century, it brought back with it a new appreciation of the sciences.

An outstanding Arab physician was known in Europe as Rhazes. An incredibly prolific writer on medical subjects, he introduced several new remedies and in about 910 AD was the first observer accurately to describe smallpox and measles as separate and distinct diseases. Another Arabian scientist, known now as Averroes (1126–1198), was the first outside Asia to recognise and record that an attack of smallpox would confer immunity to subsequent attacks.

Throughout Europe, however, the science of what we now know as epidemiology was yet to emerge. Hence, we have little idea of the actual incidence of infectious disease in the Middle Ages, in Britain or elsewhere. It is known from studies of skeletons that people suffered from leprosy and syphilis, and there are contemporary references to both leprosy and plague – but it is not clear whether the diseases these authors were describing were in fact what we now recognise as the clinical entities so named. Leprosy is from the Greek word *lepros*, which means scaly, and the term could have been applicable to any of the scores of scaling skin diseases, such as psoriasis. The word 'leprosy' is used in the Bible in a way that also makes it clear that it was a generic term, employed to cover a multitude of sicknesses. Similarly, the word 'plague' was used in the past to describe many illnesses whose only common feature was that they were all serious and could kill.

Nevertheless, true leprosy was certainly seen in Europe by the sixth century, probably being brought back from the east by returning travellers. The Knights of Saint Lazarus introduced special isolation hospitals for lepers, called 'lazarettos', or lazar houses, and one of the first of these was built in the Scilly Isles in the seventh century. Again, however, we cannot assume that all these unfortunates actually had leprosy: the word 'lazar' signifies a poor and diseased person, who may or may not have been a leper.

Bubonic plague, a major but largely undocumented scourge for uncounted ages, hit Europe with devastating ferocity in the fourteenth century.

It was called at the time 'The Great Pestilence', or 'The Great Mortality', and the evocative term 'Black Death' was not attached to this epidemic until nearly 500 years later. It is thought to have started its advance from the shores of the Black Sea in 1346, after infected Tartars catapulted their dead into a city held by besieged Genoans.

Bubonic plague is really a disease of rats, among which it is at times endemic. The plague bacillus is now known as *Yersinia pestis*. It is transferred to man by the bite of the rat flea, which is readily prepared to desert its natural host when rats become scarce in number as happens when, for example, they die of plague. During an epidemic – especially when the micro-organism invades the lungs as 'pneumonic' plague – the disease can also be transmitted from man to man in airborne droplets. It is likely also to have been directly transmitted from person to person by the human fleas which were virtually universal parasites of man during those unhygienic times. Indeed, there are dozens of types of flea known to transmit plague, just as there are hundreds of different kinds of rat that can carry them.

The animal which underpinned the disaster was the house rat, or black rat, *Rattus rattus*. This rat likes to live near people and in their homes, rather than in the open rural areas more favoured by its cousin the brown rat. It flourished in the crowded city conditions of the era, especially in the worst of the slums, and thus bubonic plague was primarily an affliction of the poor. Consequently, the distribution of the disease in Britain was very uneven. Just how many died in the Great Pestilence is not known; in the worst-affected neighbourhoods almost every person succumbed, while other localities escaped unscathed. Modern estimates of total deaths range from one-half to one-tenth of the population of Britain. According to censuses of the period, the population fell by about one-third between 1348 and 1377. Perhaps one-quarter of all the people in Europe died.

Despairing efforts were made to segregate some communities from others, and houses containing plague victims were put into isolation. It was recognised that some of the worst affected areas were around the coasts and ports, and in Italy a major maritime power, Venice, made a serious attempt to protect its people and its commerce against plague by requiring that incoming ships wait at an island in the lagoon well clear of the city for a period of thirty days. This was then extended to forty ('quaranta') days, not for what might now be regarded as rational reasons but because that period was related to the time Christ had spent in the wilderness. The system of quarantine went on to be employed by other great European seafaring cities, and to some extent is still in use today.

The Great Pestilence had profound social consequences, including diminution of the power of the Church and the dislocation of commerce. It finally demonstrated that diseases could be contagious. It marked the end of the Middle Ages and cleared the way for the Renaissance.

But bubonic plague became endemic in Britain. Indeed, celebrations of the accession of Queen Elizabeth I to the throne were curtailed because of an outbreak which killed 30,000 of her people. What was to be the last great epidemic, the Great Plague of 1665, struck London as its population escalated after the Restoration, after a quiet period which lowered the proportion of people who had been exposed non-fatally to the disease and who were thus to an extent immune. Some of the greatest writers of the age were on hand to record what they saw. Samuel Pepys, 'in great trouble' to see the weekly mortality from plague exceed 3000, wrote in August: '. . . home to draw up my will; the town growing so unhealthy, that a man cannot depend on living two days to an end. So having done something of it, to bed.'

From such writings Daniel Defoe, in his historical novel *A Journal of the Plague Year*, reconstructed in vivid terms the panic and the horror:

> . . . people sickened so fast and died so soon, that it was impossible, and indeed to no purpose, to go about to inquire who was sick and who was well . . . almost every house in a whole street being infected, and in many places every person in some of the houses; and that which was still worse, by the time that the houses were known to be infected, most of the persons known to be infected would be stone dead, and the rest run away for fear of being shut up; . . .'

However, during less dramatic times when plague grumbled on in an endemic manner, so many were the other infectious diseases besetting especially the poor, that it went almost unnoticed. Most of the other afflictions were just as untreatable and just as lethal. Names for diseases of the time can only give a clue as to what they actually were, but typhus was certainly among them. Typhus is spread by human fleas, and the customary practice of wearing the same underclothes 'from Michaelmas to Lady Day' can only have provided these parasites with every encouragement. Harvests were often bad, and famine contributed to a death toll which resulted in an average expectation of life at birth for males of about 30 years.

With leprosy and plague, the third great scourge of the Middle Ages was syphilis, the 'Great Pox'. It hardly appears in contemporary records for Britain, but it was certainly prevalent. It raced across Europe in an extraordinarily virulent form in the last years of the fifteenth century, and the fiery pattern of its spread – behaving like any other newly imported infection – supported the belief of many that this disease was brought back from the New World by Columbus' crew. There are, however, indications that a less vicious form of the disease had existed in Europe for centuries beforehand.

The behaviour of the syphilis pandemic in Europe helped to confirm the contagious nature of some diseases, but it also confirmed the belief of many theologians that diseases were punishments sent by God for sinful behaviour.

During the Renaissance, traditional dogmas were cast aside by men of towering intellect and aggressive temperament. Vesalius was one such, a man whose anatomical studies in Padua challenged the vague theories of Galen, and the Swiss Paracelsus was another, a reformer who advocated observation and experimentation as a basis for knowledge. He even went so far as to burn Galen's works in public.

Also working in Italy in the early sixteenth century was the clinician Girolamo Fracastoro ('Fracastorius'), whose written descriptions of many maladies of the time show that he recognised the specificity of the causes of disease. His major contribution came through publication in 1546 of his greatest work, *De Contagione*, in which he stated that diseases could be transmitted in three ways: by direct contact with sick people; by contact with their bedding, clothes, excreta and so on; and through the air. Each disease, he proposed, had its own *seminaria contagium*, or seed (germ). This represented the first real insight into the true nature of infectious disease. (Fracastoro also wrote a famous poem on syphilis, giving the illness its name, and we will read more of him in this context in Chapter 6.)

In Britain, a major contribution to the analysis of sickness in the community had begun at the time

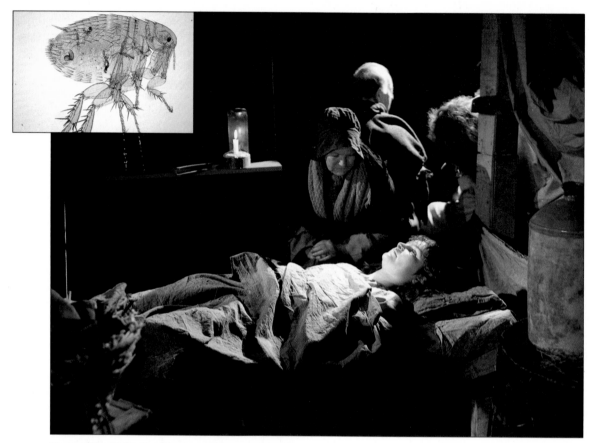

Figure 10   Bubonic plague, a disease of rats
carried to man by the flea, wiped out millions of
people throughout Europe and Asia in the Middle
Ages. At the height of the Great Plague of 1665
the weekly mortality rate rose to over 3000 in
London.

of Henry VIII with the keeping of statistical records
in the form of 'Bills of Mortality'. These comprised
data on births, deaths and disease, and were com-
piled by parish clerks on the basis of information
gathered by 'Searchers', who went to peruse the
dead and deduce the cause of death. In later years,
analysis of these figures made for powerful argu-
ments in favour of reform of appalling social
conditions.

During the seventeenth century the microscope
was first used to investigate disease, notably by the
Dutchman van Leeuwenhoek, who ground his own
lenses and constructed his own instruments. From
scrapings of his own mouth he identified bacteria.
Although it was to be 200 years before these would
be associated with the germs of disease, the theory

of contagion was soon to be vigorously promoted
by several English doctors. Among these were
Richard Mead, who maintained in 1720 that
diseased people were throwing off something that
caused contagion; Benjamin Marten, who stated
that 'animalcules' from victims of tuberculosis
would convey the disease to those who were close
to them; and Thomas Fuller, who affirmed that
particles were the cause of various 'venomous
fevers', and that different particles were specific to
the diseases that resulted.

Despite all this scientific activity (and it is worth
noting that the household names of today were
often the voices in the wilderness of yesterday), the
extent to which doctors could actually cure or
prevent infectious (or any other) disease was still

extremely limited. Bleeding, purging and cupping, often with heroic enthusiasm, were attempts to draw out evil humours and were the mainstays of treatment.

However, one of the early genuine successes was the introduction of inoculation in order to prevent smallpox, which was the most widespread fatal disease in eighteenth century Britain. This was a procedure which had been used in India and China for hundreds of years: the matter from a smallpox vesicle (the fluid-filled spot so characteristic of the disease) was transferred to a scratch on a child's skin, the resulting mild occurrence of the illness giving immunity for the rest of life. The three-year-old son of the British ambassador to Turkey was inoculated in 1718, and his wife strongly advocated the technique on her return to influential circles in London. Members of the family of George I were inoculated, and the procedure was introduced into the American colonies soon afterwards. (Centuries later, villagers in Ethiopia were robustly opposing efforts by WHO teams to stop this very same practice and replace it by something safer and more effective.)

Variolation is anything but a safe technique, and it resulted in some deaths and a few minor outbreaks of the disease despite efforts at isolation, and it was soon to be made obsolete by the work of Edward Jenner (1749–1823). He was a country general practitioner who was impressed by stories that dairymaids who had suffered from cowpox would thereafter be safe from smallpox. Cowpox is a pustular eruption of the udder of the cow, and dairymaids were prone to get similar lesions on their hands. Jenner proposed that fluid material from within these vesicles would provide protection, and in 1796 put matter from a pustule on the hand of dairymaid Sarah Nelmes into scratches in the arm of eight-year-old James Phipps. Jenner's observations were seriously flawed scientifically, but his writings stimulated work by others and the disease began to recede as an important cause of death throughout the civilised world. Just under 200 years later, smallpox was declared extinct. It was the first truly successful measure for the prevention of any infectious disease.

Infection after surgery and childbirth was at this time considered inevitable. Not all agreed that this should be so. John Burton of Edinburgh suggested in 1751 that puerperal fever might be contagious, and shortly afterwards the Manchester surgeon Charles White emphasised the need for cleanliness

in surgery and obstetrics alike. The writings of Alexander Gordon in Aberdeen also stressed what he regarded as the contagious nature of puerperal fever and, with the elegant writing of Oliver Wendell Holmes in Harvard in 1843, this proposition was brought to a wider audience. Holmes firmly maintained that a doctor who had attended upon a case of puerperal fever or erysipelas (an infectious disease of the skin) should not approach a healthy woman waiting to give birth without washing thoroughly and changing his clothes. These views were regarded at the time as highly controversial.

Coincidentally, an exceptionally controversial figure, Ignaz Semmelweiss, was making his similar views known in Europe, his strongly-expressed opinions – exceedingly unpopular with his medical colleagues – being based on his definitive observations in Vienna. However, in 1846 he was sacked from the General Hospital for his pains. Before his reinstatement the next year, a pathologist friend of his died after performing a post-

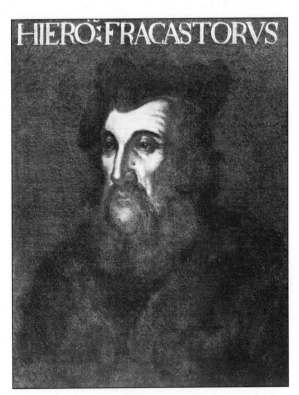

Figure 11 Fracastorius was the first to propose that disease was carried by 'germs' which could be transmitted by direct contact and through the air.

mortem examination on a victim of puerperal fever, with subsequent examination of the pathologist's body showing signs similar to those of puerperal fever. Semmelweiss concluded that 'cadaveric particles' were being carried from the post-mortem rooms by students and doctors who were then going on to examine women in labour and after birth; he insisted that all should wash their hands, and the incidence of puerperal fever dropped dramatically. Unfortunately, Semmelweiss' abrasive personality and reluctance to put his findings in writing led to his pioneering work being virtually ignored, and he died an unhappy man in 1865 – like his friend – from an infection similar to puerperal fever.

BACTERIOLOGY: A NEW SCIENCE

The founders of the science of bacteriology were Louis Pasteur (1822–1895) and Robert Koch (1843–1910), and they were the architects of what became known later as microbiology. In the late nineteenth century, the role of micro-organisms in the causation of disease was at best controversial, and at worst dismissed. Much more popular were theories on the emanations from decomposing organic matter, from toxins in the soil and from dirt generally.

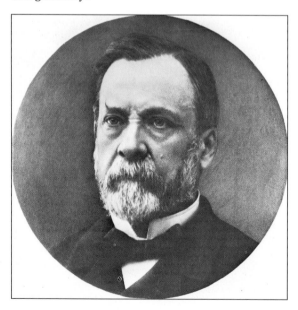

Figure 12 Louis Pasteur was one of the founders of the new science of bacteriology.

Fracastoro and others had laid the foundations for the germ theory of infectious disease some hundreds of years earlier, but had not been able to prove anything. Much weight was placed upon the competing theory of spontaneous generation, which had held since the time of Aristotle that small creatures such as grubs, flies and fleas came forth without living precursors from manure, moisture and filth. Even observation of pathogenic micro-organisms through the microscope did not prove that they caused disease.

Pasteur, like many of the most prominent scientists of the day, was a chemist. Other chemists had suggested that the process of fermentation was due to the presence of micro-organisms, and it was Pasteur who was able to prove that microbes (yeast) initiated fermentation, and that some microbes could do so in the absence of oxygen. Working for the wine industry, he showed that fermentation by contaminants could be controlled by heating ('pasteurisation'), and he went on to associate specific microbes with specific fermentations. Turning to infectious disease, Pasteur assisted the silkworm industry to locate and control a disease of these creatures which was threatening the future of silk. His studies on anthrax showed that cultures of the bacillus would produce the disease in sheep, but that germ-free filtrates would not.

He introduced the word 'vaccine' (from the Latin *vaccus*, cow) to science in honour of Edward Jenner, and his work in this field sowed the seeds for later study of the immune system. He was able to produce a vaccine for anthrax, and went on to do the same for chicken cholera and for rabies, the first successful vaccines since Jenner's vaccine for smallpox.

Pasteur's findings were in strong opposition to the doctrine of spontaneous generation, showing as they did that fermentation, the production of pus, and infectious disease all resulted from the activity of living micro-organisms.

Robert Koch was a doctor of medicine and a contemporary of Pasteur. Using simple but elegant techniques he proved that anthrax was caused by living particles which could be isolated from diseased tissue, cultured, used to re-infect other animals, and recovered again: basically, what became known as 'Koch's postulates'. He went through the same steps for tuberculosis, and isolated several other microbes in studies of infected and suppurating wounds.

The pupils and colleagues of Pasteur and Koch continued to identify new organisms as the cause of various diseases. Friedrich Loeffler and Edwin Klebs discovered the diphtheria bacillus, and a few years later Emile Roux and Alexandre Yersin demonstrated that the death dealing effects of this bacillus were due to a toxin it secreted within infected tissues. Emile von Behring showed that the serum of animals immunised by small doses of the toxin would protect other animals against its effects, which led to the first production of diphtheria antitoxin in 1896 and an almost immediate decimation of the high death rate from the disease. Thus also were further steps taken in founding the new science of immunology, a story which will be continued later in these pages.

At about the turn of the century, it was found that the agents responsible for some diseases would pass through a porcelain filter; these agents became known as 'viruses' although techniques of the time did not permit closer study of their make-up. We will pick up the story of viruses later.

With the discovery that micro-organisms caused human sickness came the belief that they might be killed without harming the humans who were their hosts, and it was another ex-colleague of Koch, Paul Ehrlich, who discovered the first specific chemical for the treatment of an infectious disease. This was the arsenical drug salvarsan, for the treatment of syphilis. The same concepts guided Ernest Fourneau, for 30 years head of the Pasteur Institute in Paris, in paving the way for the discovery of the sulphonamides and other effective antibacterial drugs. And thus, by the dawn of the twentieth century, all the seeds for the rational and successful control of infectious disease had been sown.

THE SANITARY REVOLUTION

At the beginning of the eighteenth century Britain's economy was still based on agriculture, with woollen cloth being the only export of note. Most people had enough to eat – indeed, both gross obesity and drunkenness were often dramatically depicted by painters and cartoonists of the day. But then came the wars with the French, and a succession of bad harvests. Basic foodstuffs

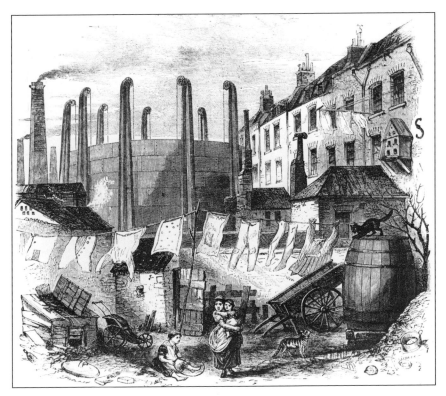

Figure 13 In the middle of the 19th century, diseases borne by sewage and water were rampant. Efforts by sanitary pioneers of the time to clean up the cities enabled epidemic diseases such as cholera to be brought under control.

became scarce and expensive, and people started migrating to the large cities such as London, Bristol and Norwich, as well as the newly-developing centres of population in the north of the country.

Smallpox had succeeded plague as the most widespread severe infectious disease, because plague – for reasons it was never possible to explain – retreated after the last great epidemic in the seventeenth century, the one which was climaxed by the great fire of London. Accompanying smallpox was epidemic typhus, which is transmitted by the human body louse and is therefore a disease of filth and crowding. During an epidemic in 1741, some one-quarter of all deaths in London were from typhus. So common was this disease in prisons it was known as 'gaol fever', and prisoners appearing at Assize courts on several occasions passed the disease on to court officers, with fatal consequences. Fifty or so gentlemen, including the Lord Mayor of London, died after trials at the Old Bailey in 1750.

Typhoid, 'enteric fever', was also endemic in the cities and a common way to die. Infantile diarrhoea, like typhoid probably resulting from contamination of water supplies, caused a high rate of fatal illness, especially in the summer months. Throat infections, including diphtheria and scarlet fever, caused havoc among children and were a frequent cause of death, and tuberculosis and epidemic influenza added to the total count of fatal illness whose spread was made easy by crammed and dirty conditions. Medicine, at the time, had nothing to offer. Under the existing living conditions, the prospects for a long and successful life for the lethal microbes were much better than for the human beings who suffered such a terrible toll.

As the year 1800 passed, things got worse. The population increased rapidly, and industrialisation drew people to the mushrooming new industrial towns in the provinces. Rows upon rows of cramped terraces were thrown together, in an attempt to house the burgeoning population, by local authorities without the faintest notion of the principles of town planning or public hygiene. Contemporary descriptions of conditions in the provincial towns of the industrial revolution tell in evocative fashion of defective or non-existent drainage, of cesspools and privies – open within the houses – draining through open gutters into the streets, and of open slaughter-houses where offal was left to rot. Nightsoil collectors built festering piles of dung in their backyards. Chamber-pots were dumped in the roadway, and buckets of nightsoil were tossed from upper stories with the shout of 'gardy loo!'. This, as one writer observed laconically, was inconvenient for the passer by, and the more prosperous took to travelling in the security of closed coaches and sedan chairs.

The places of work were no better, and the rural poor also lived in squalor. The general level of nutrition was pretty terrible, based as it was on bread and potatoes, and water supplies were limited in quantity and polluted. Typhus, cholera and tuberculosis were the main causes of death at the dawn of the age of Queen Victoria.

Cholera was endemic only in India and the Far East until the eighteenth century, when travellers along the great trade routes of the world started moving it west. It became the classic epidemic disease of the nineteenth century. The first pandemic, of 1817 to 1823, spared Europe, but the second did not. It finally reached Britain, whose inhabitants had anxiously tracked it across the European continent, in late 1831. From the port of Sunderland it raced north to Scotland and south through England, Wales and Ireland, killing some 60,000 people and concentrating on the poorer and more densely-populated areas.

Responsibility for the care of the poor rested with local administrative bodies, often disorganised and corrupt. While it was accepted that appalling living and working conditions were at least partly responsible for poor health, the argument was whether to apportion available funds to the care of sick people or to 'nuisances' such as streets flowing with sewage. Charles Dickens, in *Oliver Twist*, wrote of Southwark thus:

> '. . . a maze of close, narrow and muddy streets . . . Crazy wooden galleries common to the backs of half-a-dozen houses, with holes from which to look upon the slime beneath . . . rooms so small, so filthy and squalor which they shelter . . . dirt-besmeared walls and decaying foundations; every repulsive lineament of poverty, every loathsome indication of filth, rot and garbage.'

Several of the more favoured citizens blamed both the poverty and the poor health on lack of moral fibre and intemperance; the 'profligacy and drunkenness of the lower orders' was a matter for 'public remark' and censure.

But the horrors of the cholera epidemic forced a demand for more effective action. The Poor Laws were reviewed in 1832, and Poor Law Commissioners were appointed to direct the central office which, in turn, was to allocate responsibility for necessary changes to local government bodies. Edwin Chadwick was appointed Secretary to the Commissioners, one of the best appointments in the history of public administration.

Chadwick was a lawyer who had worked as a journalist during his training and was therefore exceptionally good at gathering, condensing and preparing understandable information for distribution to a wide audience. He was also a close associate of other liberal reformers. These included John Stuart Mill and a doctor who spent his life trying to improve conditions for the poor, Dr Thomas Southwood Smith. Smith's own angry reports to Parliament were freely quoted in the fictional material of his friend Charles Dickens.

Chadwick's landmark paper, *Report on the Sanitary Condition of the Labouring Population of Great Britain* (1842), shone a glaring spotlight on the conditions of the time. It included a careful analysis of the most important causes of death – 'consumption', typhus and scarlet fever – and pinpointed their distribution. He concentrated in his report on the inadequate sewage disposal which resulted in such unspeakable squalor, and suggested that contaminated sources of drinking water were a threat to health.

Chadwick's report stimulated the formation of a Royal Commission, followed by the Factory Act of 1847 (to regulate the hours and conditions of work for women and children) and the Act for Promoting Public Health, which was passed by Parliament in 1848. This Act was to prove as important a part of preventive medicine as anything done by the bacteriologists; indeed, Chadwick did not even believe in the germ theory of disease. Inspectors were sent out to investigate and report on sewerage, drainage, water supplies, burial grounds, street lighting and surfacing. Local boards of health were established, liaising with the central commissioners, and this pattern was to be the model for subsequent similar moves in the United States.

However, and unfortunately for Chadwick, he was as abrasive in his personal relationships as many other pioneers in public health, and he was finally dismissed – not that this prevented his continuing to influence Parliament with his writings.

In 1836 the Births and Deaths Registration Act was passed, and Chadwick used his influence to

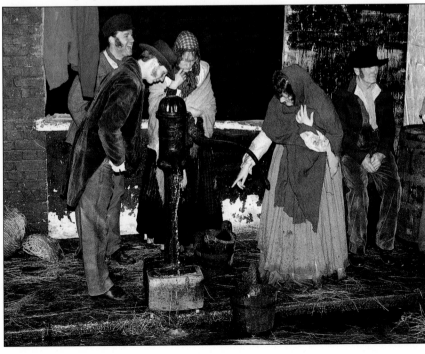

Figure 14 The cause of the 1854 epidemic of cholera in London was infected water from the public pump in Broad Street, Soho.

have Dr William Farr appointed to administer it. Farr was a superb statistician, and it was he who analysed data relating to life and death in Britain in such a way that Chadwick could make the best possible public use of it. Another influential man to make good use of Farr's figures was the first Medical Officer of Health for the City of London, Sir John Simon, a surgeon from St Thomas' Hospital, who was appointed to his public position in 1848. He proved to be an outstanding administrator, less combative than Chadwick and able to bridge the gap between the engineers and the medical practitioners.

Another protégé of Chadwick's, Dr John Snow, was to be one of the first to demonstrate the fallacy of the belief of his mentor – and almost all others – that diseases arose from filth and were spread by miasmas. Cholera continued to sweep across Britain, with three epidemics causing terrible losses in a space of 20 years. During the epidemic of 1854 Snow plotted the location of cases of cholera on a map of London, and saw that there was a concentration round a public water pump in Broad Street, Soho. He had the handle of the pump removed and the epidemic, as it happened already on the decline, ceased soon afterwards. He went on to use Farr's data to compare the incidence of cholera in houses with different water supplies, and showed that water coming from cleaner supplies further up the Thames was associated with a much lower rate of cholera. His conclusion: 'Diseases that are communicated from person to person are caused by some material which passes from the sick to the healthy, and which has the property of increasing and multiplying in the system of the person it attacks.'

Dr William Budd came to a similar conclusion in the case of typhoid, which at the time was also thought to be spread through the air in some vaporous manner. He was the only doctor in the village of North Tawton, near Bristol, and carried out careful epidemiological studies very similar to those of Snow. He concluded in a paper published in 1856 that the principal means of spread was by contamination of drinking water by the excreta of the sick. (The next year Budd correctly suggested that tuberculosis was spread by specific germs in the sputum of sufferers.) His studies, and those of Snow, thus proved the germ theory of disease long before the bacteriological studies of Pasteur and Koch finally put the matter to rest.

So, as the nineteenth century drew to an end, living conditions in Britain were improving in such a way that the risk of infectious disease was lower, thanks largely to the efforts of the sanitary pioneers. Houses were cleaner, lighter, better ventilated; water supplies were more abundant and cleaner; and sewerage systems were disposing of a greater proportion of sewage. There were sharp falls in the incidence of typhus and typhoid, and cholera and smallpox were disappearing. Tuberculosis was still a dreaded disease, however, and conditions of work remained poor.

In the United States, a book dealer called Lemuel Shattuck was emulating what Chadwick was trying to accomplish in Britain, and after reporting highly unfavourably on the state of sanitation in Massachusetts, stimulated efforts for the establishment of a State Board of Health. Other States quickly followed suit. At the federal level, the new American Public Health Service took over quarantine functions from the individual ports.

THE LEGACY OF NIGHTINGALE

Nursing orders were established under the Catholic Church as a result of the needs generated by the wars of the Crusades. They included the Knights of St John, the Teutonic Knights, and the Knights of Lazarus. Corresponding orders for women were established, and through charity, nurses working at hospitals for the indigent sick throughout Europe did a great service for the poor.

However, in the countries whose church organisations were overthrown by the Reformation nursing fell into some decline, although in Ireland the Sisters of Charity and the Sisters of Mercy kept the flame alive.

Florence Nightingale was a well-born lady with a burning, life-long desire to improve the conditions of care for the sick. After early work – which she denied was 'training' – in a Protestant monastery in Germany and various Catholic institutions in Paris, she returned to London and developed her pioneering ideas on nursing administration. In order to obtain further information for the promotion of her crusade, she made her famous trip to the Crimean War. On her return to England a grateful public raised enough money for the establishment of the first school of nursing at St Thomas' Hospital in 1860, and her books and her influence established nursing as a career of status and skill.

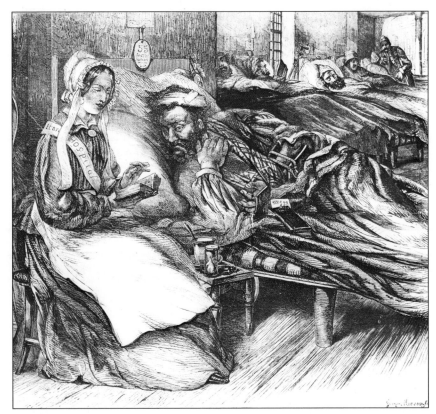

Figure 15 The strenuous efforts of Florence Nightingale and her successors brought cleanliness to the care of patients and a reduction in infectious disease.

Schools of nursing were soon thereafter established in the United States.

In her *Notes on Nursing: What it is and what it is not* (1859) Florence Nightingale offered advice on hygiene in the home, the need for thorough cleanliness when caring for the young, the sick and the aged, and on healthy diet and storage of food and milk products. She provided guidance on the decorating and furnishing of houses, on the clothing of children and on the prevention of the spread of infection. In the foreword to the 1952 edition of this book the then President of the Royal College of Nursing stated '. . . her book must have done as much to prevent sickness and accidents in English homes than any other influence of the time'. Her reforming zeal was to influence political decisions for the rest of her century, and her ideas are still relevant to the control of infection today.

MODERN TIMES AND THE WORLD HEALTH ORGANISATION

Although nations and city states such as Venice had been moved to local action in attempts to keep particular epidemics from their walls, international cooperation for centuries played no part whatsoever in efforts to prevent infectious diseases spreading. But the repeated sweeps of cholera across an increasingly anxious Europe forced a change. In Paris in late 1851 the French convened what was to be the first of a series of international sanitary conferences, starting with the gathering that year attended by 11 European countries, and ending with the fourteenth in 1938, at which 50 countries from all around the world were represented.

In the early days cholera was the main focus of discussion, but the epidemiological studies of those such as Snow were largely ignored. Even though the 1874 conference was prepared to agree that drinking water could cause disease, the views of those who did not believe in contagion generally prevailed. Indeed, the British representatives insisted – and continued to insist through the conferences of 1881 and 1885 – that cholera could not be passed from person to person. This official position was politically rather than scientifically motivated: all the other European countries maintained (correctly) that the reservoirs for cholera were to be found in India, but the British perceived that to accept this as being so, together with the concept of contagion, would pose a serious threat to trade with their important colony. It was not until 1892 that the British representative was able to state that his Government now agreed with everyone else – and thus, implicitly, with Snow's proof of transmission published 39 years previously. By the end of the century, therefore, it was possible for international agreements to be reached on the movement of ships from east to west and on the official notification of cholera outbreaks world wide.

In 1902 the American States formed what was to become the Washington-based Pan American Sanitary Bureau, and in Europe a permanent body, the Office International d'Hygiene Publique, was established in Paris five years later. This office supplied information to the international sanitary conferences and entered into liaison with the Health Organisation of the League of Nations in 1919. The United States was not a member of the League, but provided substantial support through the Rockefeller Foundation, whose Institute for Medical Research (founded in 1901) was later to make outstanding international contributions to the control of infectious disease.

In 1943 the Allied nations signed an agreement to establish the United Nations Relief and Rehabilitation Agency (UNRRA), with the purpose (among others) of preventing epidemic disease among refugees and liberated populations. A huge programme was launched after the war, concentrating on the control of diphtheria with antitoxin, blocking the spread of typhus and malaria with DDT, and controlling at a global level cholera, tuberculosis and sexually transmitted diseases.

The 1945 meeting which established the United Nations appeared temporarily to have disregarded health, bowed down as it was by weightier issues, but three years later the World Health Organisation was born. Its basic strategy, established then and continuing, is to provide advice and information to all countries about problems affecting the health of the public. Its presently defined goal is to make possible the attainment of 'Health for All by the year 2000'. From the earliest days its emphasis was on the control of infectious diseases, and this has continued because they still have such a devastating effect on millions of people throughout the world, especially in the developing countries. Even today, one of the major obstacles to the achievement of the organisation's monumental goal is the explosive growth in incidence of an infectious disease not even recognised a few years ago, AIDS.

The richer nations have used scientific knowledge and enlightened public administration (and a great deal of money) to combat the 'nuisances' which cause infection; but in the rest of the world, the nuisances – filth, poverty, malnutrition and appalling housing – remain.

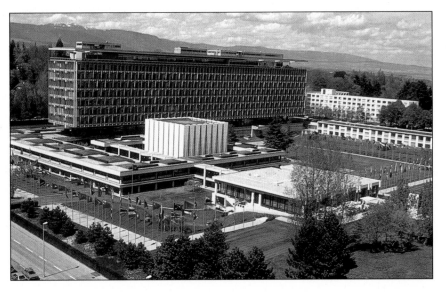

Figure 16 The World Health Organisation, with its headquarters in Geneva, provides advice and information to all countries about problems affecting the health of the public.

CHAPTER

3

Patterns of Infection

A TORRENT OF CHANGE

Following the work of the sanitary pioneers, there has been a remarkable change in patterns of mortality since early Victorian times, from the darker side of which we have drawn such a gloomy picture. Among children and adolescents in Britain the death rate (standardised for changes in age and sex distribution over the years) is now less than one-tenth of that which prevailed in the mid-1800s. For those aged in their sixties, the death rate has been about halved, and for the oldest age group it has fallen by about one-third. Over the same period the number of babies dying soon after birth has fallen from one in seven to one in seventy-seven.

Nearly half of all the human beings who died in Victorian times were children. Now, only about one in fifty of all deaths occur between birth and the age of 14 years.

So, what has happened is that although for those who survive childhood there is no great promise of a vastly extended term of life – the Biblical three score years and ten are still not that far from the mark – there has been an enormous increase in the proportion of those who are born who will live

through their childhood and still be alive 50 or 70 years later. It is this 'bulge' in the middle years of life that has so improved life expectancy on average.

The main reason for this change is that there has been a striking reduction in infectious disease as a cause of death in all age groups. Because younger people were never in the first place so likely to die from non-infectious conditions such as cancer and diseases of the circulation, the improvement has been relatively much greater for them. Because of the decline in the relative importance of infectious disease as a cause of death among the young, it is now accidents and violence which are the single most important cause of death until well into the fourth decade of life.

The character of infectious disease in the community, therefore, has changed in two main ways: in its incidence, and in its duration. Not only are fewer people becoming infected, but when that does happen, it is for a shorter time and probably with fewer unpleasant consequences. Healing can be achieved more rapidly than in past years. The killer infections are not at present a significant factor in mortality statistics in Britain and similar countries, and the scene is now dominated by short-lived and acute but benign infections, most of them caused by viruses.

Over the millennia, pathogenic micro-organisms have necessarily adopted a strategy which allows them to survive and prosper but without destroying their hosts, because without them they cannot survive either. So, as some relationships become longstanding ones, the virulence of the surviving pathogens tends to diminish. At the same time, their hosts are selecting from their population individuals who are more resistant to the ill effects of the pathogens. Hence, the feature of these long-standing relationships is the stability which has evolved, to which we referred in the opening chapter.

However, over recent decades, many such long-standing relationships have not been allowed to persist in a rapidly evolving community, because of man's inclination for making rapid changes to his environment and his way of life. Adaptations have simply not had time to happen. Thus, the interaction of pathogenic organisms and particular communities has been affected more by new outside influences than by gradual evolutionary changes. The recent and highly favourable transformations in the pattern of infectious disease which we have seen as history unfolds have not generally been because of fundamental alterations either in the infecting organisms or in man himself. It is technology and the environment which have changed. Organisms grown on culture media have shown no basic change in their potential to infect human beings; the new factor is that our power to identify organisms has brought a whole range of organisms freshly to our notice. Even organisms which have shown a remarkable capacity to circumvent our best efforts at preventing their onslaught by shifts in their antigens, such as the influenza virus, have not thereby changed to any significant extent their danger to us as pathogens. Man's basic powers of resistance are the same as they have been since observation began, and so are his immunological mechanisms.

What has changed is the extent to which we are now able to influence micro-organisms themselves, the response of the human body to them, and the environment in which the pathogens and man are living. In terms of technical equipment, what is now available to medicine is, first, a far greater precision of diagnosis, being the detection and differentiation of disease; second, the availability of the science of immunology, and the use of prophylactic immunisation; and, third, more effective therapy, which has improved the control of individual cases of disease. The result of all this is that infectious diseases are now less prevalent; they are responsible for fewer deaths; and as a general rule they are less likely to have fatal consequences.

At the same time, however, as we manipulate the environment in order to reduce the contact between man and microbe, we make inevitable a greater risk of worse disease when contact does occur, because we are reducing the opportunity for resistance to build up in the early years of life. Paradoxically, therefore, the more successful that our attempts at prevention are in the present, the more essential it becomes to ensure that they remain successful in the future.

As we have suggested, the distribution of infectious diseases throughout the population is very different from what it was (and fortunately for us, too — we would hardly be content with what our Victorian forebears suffered). However, our continuing predilection for squeezing together in urban conglomerations means that infections spread by droplets and by close and intimate contact are as common as ever. Indeed, the rate of spread of an infection within a community is a function of the number of sources of the disease and the number of susceptible hosts who come into contact with it, and both these factors are inevitably influential when an infection is introduced into an urban community.

'New' diseases: legionellosis and Lassa fever

Populations which have not been living with particular pathogens lose their resistance to them as time goes by, and if they have never been exposed to them they can have built up no resistance at all. This may be of particular importance in the case of the occasional but regular introduction of diseases which are 'new' to Britain, three recent and well-known examples being Legionnaires' disease, acquired immune deficiency syndrome (AIDS) and Lassa fever. AIDS we will consider in more detail later, in the context of diseases which can be transmitted by sexual intercourse, but the other two of these illnesses are both instructive examples of how previously unrecognised conditions can change our appreciation of patterns of disease.

In July 1976, members of the American Legion ('Legionnaires') attended a convention at a large hotel in Philadelphia. An explosive outbreak of pneumonia hit the delegates, and also affected some other citizens of the city. Dozens of them died. But the cause of the pneumonia was a mystery, and remained so for nearly six months. The reason turned out to be that the organism was a small bacterium which was very hard to stain with a dye so that it could be seen under the microscope, and it was also very hard to persuade to grow on culture media. Once unmasked, it was found (from testing of materials preserved from earlier unexplained outbreaks of pneumonia) that it must have been around for a very long time, but hitherto unrecognised.

Not only was it hard to see or grow, it was highly unusual in its ability to live quite happily separately from man or any other organic home base. The organism, now known as *Legionella pneumophila*, colonises hot and cold water systems, including bathroom shower heads and air-conditioning cooling towers and condensers. It has also been found in natural creeks, ponds, and the mud from their banks. It spreads in droplets of water, but apparently only very rarely from person to person.

It has gained the reputation of being a 'killer germ' because of its often well-publicised identification following fatal outbreaks of pneumonia, but it is really no more likely to be lethal than any other organism which causes pneumonia. Indeed, it has probably been causing pneumonia for many years – cases back to 1947 have been proved to be a result of it – but generally without fatal consequences, and it is now accepted that it must always have been a common cause of the condition. About 200 cases are reported each year in England and Wales. It causes about 3% of all pneumonias, and previously healthy and fit young people are unlikely to suffer anything more than a minor illness. However, the elderly, and especially smokers, are at greater risk, and the mortality rate among such groups is in the order of 15%. It tends to be thought of as a travellers' disease, but this is because the most publicised outbreaks have occurred among groups staying in air-conditioned hotels. In fact, it occurs in all countries of the world, and there are so many slightly different varieties of the organism now being found that the disease is better known as 'legionellosis'.

The relevance of legionellosis to the present discussion is that it apparently emerged as a new disease but was later shown to have been around for a long time unrecognised – basically because

we had never thought of looking for such bacteria in the places it liked to live. As far as mankind was concerned, the organism was living harmlessly in mud and water until environmental changes brought it out, planted it in cooling towers and air-conditioning plants, and came then to regard it as a 'pathogen'. We cannot tell how many other such discoveries there may be in the future.

Lassa fever is different from legionellosis in that it is really very rare in the developed world, but similar in that it seemed to be 'new' when it appeared. It was first recognised when hospital staff attending patients with an unexplained fever succumbed to serious illness, and it has since achieved a status of considerable notoriety. Lassa fever is caused by a virus which is distributed quite widely in Africa, especially in rural areas. People returning from Africa with an unexplained fever are far more likely to be suffering from malaria than Lassa fever, but its high mortality rate (about 15% of patients admitted to hospital with the disease) and the fact that hospital staff are among the most likely people to be infected by the patient, make it a disease which is handled very warily indeed. Indeed, proven cases are strictly isolated. This, then, is another disease which is new to countries outside Africa, from where travellers can unwittingly bring it, and against which we have to be on our guard.

Not only are 'new' diseases emerging on the scene, but also 'new' pathogens are being identified, to which we can relate known illnesses with previously unknown causes. 'Non-specific' urethritis, a sexually-transmitted disease, got that name because its cause was unknown. Now, it is clear that the majority of cases are due to an organism called *Chlamydia*, which we have recognised as being around for a long time, but in different connections; and other causes for the condition are also being discovered. Much enteritis of 'unknown' aetiology is now known to arise from the effects of viruses such as rotaviruses, and infectious diarrhoea from the effects of bacteria such as *Campylobacter*.

The point of this is to show that organisms which are new to us are continually being isolated and associated with clinical disease, and that many diseases of presently unknown aetiology may well turn out to be of infectious origin. Thus, the relative part recorded as being played by infection in future death and morbidity statistics may look a little different from now. We must remain on the

Expectation of age at death, 1841–1981

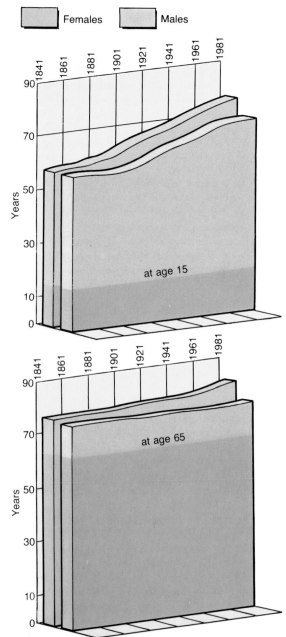

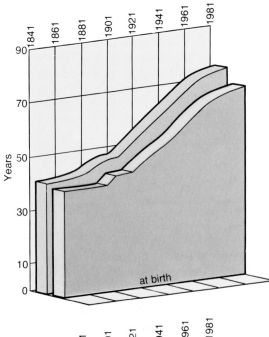

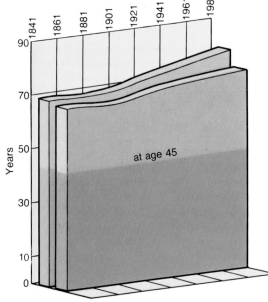

Figure 17   Most of the improvement in life expectancy has been due to greatly reduced death rates in the very young. The figure shows that a man could expect to live to the age of 35 when born in 1841, but to 70 when born in 1981. The life expectancy of a man aged 65 has not changed much during the same period, although it has improved a little for women.
(Source: Office of Population Censuses and Surveys).

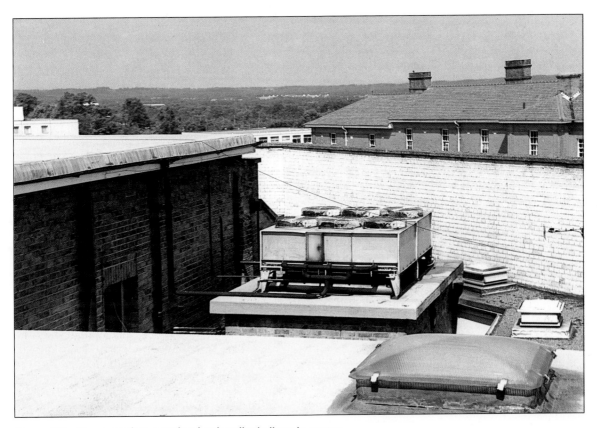

Figure 18   The organism causing Legionellosis lives in water and thrives in the air-conditioning cooling towers of modern buildings.

lookout. If we do not watch, we will not see.

Maintaining control

Because in modern times we seem to have virtually eliminated infection as a significant factor in mortality, there is a danger that complacency will cause us to place too much reliance on drugs, doctors and pesticides to keep it under control. There is plenty of scope for breakdown in the complex system we have built to protect ourselves from serious infectious disease, and we will describe examples of how this can happen in more detail at appropriate places later in this book. They will include breakdowns in immunisation status of the community, breakdowns in the way we try to keep diseases from being imported, and breakdowns in the way we try to ensure pure food and uncontaminated water. The present favourable pattern of infectious disease in nations such as Britain will only continue if we make positive efforts, not only medical and scientific ones, but also at a personal level.

At present, however, most preventable infectious disease in the community continues to exist because of deficiencies in the application or enforcement of control measures. In some parts of Britain, and in many less prosperous parts of the world, infectious disease continues because the resistance of individual human beings has been compromised by poverty and malnutrition; the old triad of famine, war and pestilence still plays its part in the affairs of mankind. Even in the developed world, stress, alcohol and drugs can place individuals in a poor position to fight off infection. Hence, among the major defences against communicable diseases today must be included economic development and the promotion of physical and mental health.

INFECTIONS TODAY

In industrialised western countries there has been a tremendous drop in rates of death from infectious disease during the present century, with some dramatic falls in deaths from some particular diseases. For example, diphtheria and acute polio-myelitis have been almost eradicated. Today, the total number of deaths (in absolute terms) from infectious disease in Britain is between one-quarter and one-third of the figure for 1940; and, expressed as a percentage of all deaths in the last 50 years, the proportion has dropped from some 20% to around 3%.

As indicated in the discussion on changing patterns of mortality, it is the diseases which used particularly to strike at children that have been subject to the most dramatic drops. For instance, the number of reported cases of measles in 1951 was 636,000, and in 1986 it was 90,000, a drop of some seven times.

It is quite easy to measure deaths, because of accurate diagnosis and reporting, but it is a good deal harder to measure the incidence of morbi-dity – non-fatal illness – within any community, even developed ones. Statistics for notifiable and non-fatal infectious disease are gathered, however, and in Britain are published by the various census offices on the basis of collation by communicable disease surveillance centres.

Recent changes in morbidity can be attributed at least in part to the use of pharmaceutical agents, and of these it has been the vaccines used in immunisation programmes which have had the most dramatic effect. Poliomyelitis, a disease once much dreaded because of the risk of paralysis following it, has been almost wiped out in Europe, the United States and Canada. In the developing countries, by way of sad contrast, little or no protective cover from immunisation has been provided until recently, and indeed during the 1960s there was a clear increase in the incidence of polio in Africa, Asia and Latin America, with the number of cases rising rapidly from what had been a low base rate.

The use of measles vaccine, similarly, has shown that the disease can be eradicated, an aim which is justified because of the risk of brain damage among a proportion of the children who get the disease. However, the incidence in some countries – inclu-ding the United States – has recently been edging

up again, as people's perception of measles as a serious risk to health drops as a result of the disease itself dropping from public notice. In tropical countries measles tends to arise in a more virulent form, with a high risk of complications, and the need for widespread immunisation – in many places unmet – is even greater.

Whooping cough is a potentially serious illness in children, and is one of those which is subject to mass immunisation programmes in the developed world. As a result, great reductions in incidence have become apparent. Again, however, rates of immunisation vary from year to year, a pheno-menon fuelled in part by a public awareness that there is a tiny risk of complications following the procedure, an awareness which is much more acute than that awakened by the greater risk to the community as a whole of complications following the illness. In the United Kingdom notifications of whooping cough dropped rapidly between 1951 and 1961, but there have been occasional surges in incidence since then, especially apparent in the 1985–86 period, with nearly 40,000 cases notified.

In the case of rubella (German measles) the policy in Britain is to offer immunisation to girls and susceptible women, and in 1985, 86% of schoolgirls were immunised against rubella by the age of 14 years.

For the less serious childhood diseases, such as chickenpox, while immunisation is in principle possible, it is not considered worth the small risk except for a few people with deficiencies of their immune systems. Accordingly, the incidence of these diseases has remained about the same over the years.

Meningitis caused by the 'meningococcus' (Neisseria meningitidis) was once quite common in Europe, and after a period during which it was virtually unknown it is now staging a comeback. Notifications of acute meningitis in Britain showed a large increase of 39% between 1985 and 1986, rising to 2,500 cases, most of the increase being due to acute meningococcal meningitis, with 858 cases notified. In 1987, 1090 cases of meningococcal meningitis with 158 deaths were reported, mostly among children. The local nature of many out-breaks of the infection causes understandable alarm among parents, and this is one of the few cases in which it may be desirable to use an anti-biotic as a preventive measure for the families and close contacts of the infected.

Erysipelas and other infections caused by the

streptococci, such as sore throats and scarlet fever, have practically disappeared in the developed world, not only because of the introduction of antibiotics but also because of a diminution in the virulence of the responsible organisms apparent during the present century. The incidence of syphilis and gonorrhoea showed a marked decrease with the introduction of antibiotics into general use, but rose again after the 1950s. This trend has been reversed to some extent in recent years, along with changes in sexual behaviour associated with the fear of AIDS. However, non-specific venereal diseases which are not primarily bacterial — genital warts, genital herpes and non-specific urethritis — are on the increase.

Some infectious diseases have shown little change over the years. In particular, respiratory infections remain a serious problem to people in the developed and undeveloped world alike. There are plenty of drugs now available to kill bacteria, but over 90% of acute respiratory infections are caused by viruses, against which drugs are still practically all ineffective. Further, smoking is known to affect the tissue of the lungs in such a way that invasion by respiratory pathogens becomes more likely and more dangerous. No one is a stranger to respiratory infections, so the misery they can cause is well known to all, and they are responsible for considerable economic losses from the number of days they cause people to be off work. Respiratory illnesses account for about one-third of all absences from work and school in Britain. The influenza virus, one of the world's most successful parasites, still takes an impressive toll of lives world wide.

Among other groups of diseases showing little change in incidence are the various food poisoning syndromes and viral hepatitis.

Tuberculosis has continued the steady decline in Britain which has accompanied rising living standards. It is now a disease virtually confined to the elderly and to immigrant people.

The picture in the developing world is very different from that in the industrialised nations. The WHO has estimated that whereas throughout the developed world some 8% of all deaths are from infectious disease, the equivalent figure for the developing world is nearly 40%, divided evenly between respiratory infections and all others, including diarrhoea. Because of the much greater number of people in the developing world, the net effect is that infectious diseases still cause about one-third of all fatal diseases, world wide. It is in the third world where the fight continues against the great epidemic diseases which have figured so strongly throughout history, and typhus and yellow fever have at last been contained within very small areas. Smallpox, of course, has been totally eliminated. In temperate climates at least, malaria is under better control than it used to be, although once-high hopes for its world-wide eradication have now been abandoned. However, the incidence of much less dramatic infectious illnesses, such as diarrhoea in infants – perhaps today's greatest single killer of all – remains sickeningly high. Also very far from control in many areas are diseases caused by parasitic protozoa and helminths, and in some places the incidence of the diseases they cause is still rising.

Figure 19 Graphs show the marked decrease in the rate of important infectious diseases between 1948 and 1987.
* Provisional.
(Source: Office of Population Censuses and Surveys, and Statistical Review).

Polio

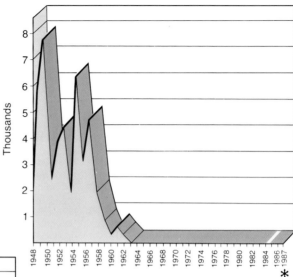

Scarlet fever

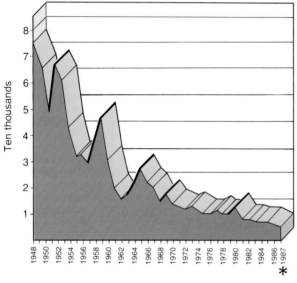

Measles

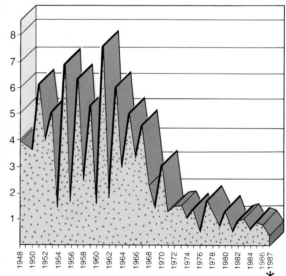

CHAPTER

4

The Microbes, Helminths and Fungi

THE MICROBES

Having discussed the history, changing patterns and present incidence of infectious disease, we now turn to more detailed examination of the microorganisms which are responsible. For a while, accordingly, the spotlight falls on the microbes rather than the illness they cause.

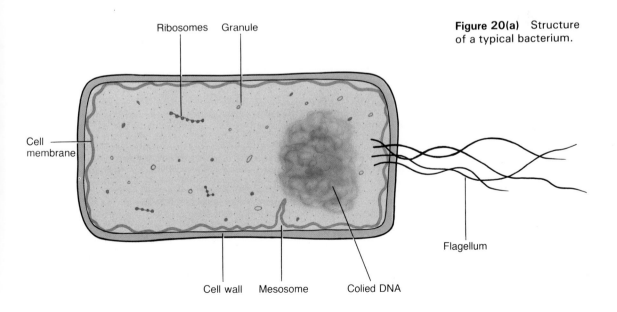

Figure 20(a) Structure of a typical bacterium.

Ribosomes   Granule

Cell membrane

Cell wall   Mesosome   Colied DNA

Flagellum

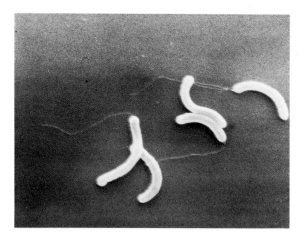

Figure 20(b)   Scanning electron micrograph of Vibrio Cholerae; (magnification × 8,000).

In doing so, however, we should bear in mind that in the western world there is a move away from relating specific, named micro-organisms to specific, named diseases. This is still a wholly valid association in poorer countries, where the traditional fevers such as malaria, tuberculosis, yellow fever, cholera, plague and so on are still of epidemiological importance, but it oversimplifies the situation for the infections most commonly seen elsewhere.

Following Koch's discoveries, it was perfectly understandable for medical scientists to aim their countermeasures at the specific microbes which they discovered in patients who were ill. However, as we have commented earlier, we are sharing the world with a huge variety of micro-organisms, many of which are parasitic on humans, but only a small proportion of which do actually cause disease. There exists, therefore, a spectrum of disease-causing ability, from very nasty to quite benign, and when a person becomes ill it is not always possible to assign the cause to one particular germ. Indeed, we are still finding 'new' microbes, such as *Legionella*, which were there all the time (probably) but which we had no idea could cause pneumonia.

And pneumonia is an example of how one illness can be caused by perhaps dozens of different organisms and environmental factors, some of which we may know about and some of which we may not. The same applies to infections of the urinary tract, alimentary canal and respiratory system. Babies dying from the dehydration caused by diarrhoea in refugee camps may be found to have an incredible variety of pathogenic organisms swarming all over them, but they may still be saved not by killing particular organisms but rather by being given replacement fluids to drink.

Nevertheless, along with the development of practical ways of treating disease has come a fascination by scientists with the intrinsic characteristics of the responsible organisms, leading to discoveries on the fundamental chemistry of living things. Such studies have been refined over the years right down to the molecular level, and our understanding of the synthesis of protein, with all its implications, sprang originally from the study of bacteria and viruses.

The three great groups of organisms responsible for most of the infectious disease in man in the western world are the bacteria, the viruses, and the protozoa. In the warmer and poorer countries these may be matched or surpassed in importance by fungi and by worms (helminths)—see Appendix B.

Bacteria

Pretty well everyone has some basic idea of what bacteria look like. They are composed of one cell only, and occur in three main forms: spherical, called cocci; rod-like, known as bacilli; and spiral. Many of them can move around on their own in fluid, using hairs (flagella).

They are very small, being measured in microns (thousandths of a millimetre), but with considerable variations in size. The small *Haemophilus influenzae*, for example, is only about half a micron long by one-fifth of a micron wide; *Bacillus anthracis*, at the other extreme, may be ten microns in length. The electron microscope shows that each bacterium has a rigid cell wall which provides support and protection for the cell membrane, the living surface of the organism. It is the way the cell wall is built up which determines the antigenic properties of the bacterium, and hence the immune response to its invasion. It also determines the response to some antibiotic drugs. A few can develop hard-shelled spores within their cell walls in response to unfavourable environmental conditions, and in this form – resistant to heat, drying out, and chemicals – they can survive.

Bacteria multiply for the most part by splitting in the middle: 'binary fission'. As we have already commented, they can do this at astonishing speed, and several pounds of dried bacteria can easily be obtained just by letting them get on with it under controlled conditions. The typical time between each division is 20 minutes, so that under unrealistically perfect conditions a bacterium weighing one-millionth of a gram will have produced progeny weighing over a kilogram within seven hours, multiplying to one million kilograms (about a thousand tons) in the same time again. This cannot actually happen; but it does show how fast bacteria can multiply in, say, contaminated food, or in the absence of any defensive mechanisms in the body to stop them.

Each individual division is supposed to result in precise replication of the cell DNA – but during the billions of divisions that take place, things occasionally go slightly wrong. A change in the DNA means mutation. Most mutations lead to the death of the organisms, but just once in a while the mutation means that the organism is better able to cope with the conditions of the environment in which it finds itself at the time. So, that particular organism thrives – and, as it multiplies, the number of those which are thriving grows faster than the others and the bacterium 'evolves'. This is, of course, the same as happens in the wider world, but a lot more slowly. In part, this amazingly rapid evolution explains how bacteria can 'adapt' to their environment, and to chemicals that are sent to destroy them.

Bacteria, like any other living organisms, require nutrients to live on; but unlike garden plants they contain no chlorophyll which they could use to obtain energy. Most bacteria that thrive in the world around us live in any kind of decaying organic matter, from which they obtain their food; indeed, their main function in nature is to break down such matter into the simple substances that can be used by plants and thus, indirectly – through the food chain – by animals. To help such breakdown is the whole point of building a compost heap.

Other bacteria obtain their nutrients from the bodies of living animals. The digestive tract is packed with billions of bacteria – in fact, they make up about half the bulk of the faeces – and others find a contented living on our skin, especially where it is moist and damp, or in the mucous membranes which line (among other places) the mouth, nose and throat. But it is only when they turn to surviving at the expense of the living cells around them that they can cause illness.

The bacteria called 'cocci' group together in characteristic ways. Staphylococci, for example, form bunches, like the grapes which give them their name. Streptococci are strung together in strings.

Staphylococci occur in three species, two of which are pretty harmless while the other is not: *Staphylococcus aureus*, or 'golden staph'. Staphylococci are carried by humans who are perfectly well, and they are particularly likely to be found within the nose. People who work in hospitals are mere mortals, and as such they can also carry pathogenic staph in their noses; in which instance they can carry the organisms to individuals who are sick or otherwise vulnerable. Studies have shown that around 40% of healthy hospital personnel may be carrying these organisms in their noses and throats. Similarly pathogenic strains of staph can be cultured from the hands of healthy people, and it is difficult to get rid of these even by the vigorous scrubbing which precedes surgery.

The main obvious effect of infection by staphylococci is the production of pus: boils, abscesses and suppurating wounds. But staph also produce toxins of great lethality. A well-publicised but rare example is the 'toxic shock' which was suffered by women using a vaginal tampon which had become colonised by certain strains of *Staphylococcus aureus*. These produced a toxin that was responsible for the illness. If staphylococcal toxins get into the blood, a lethal variety of blood poisoning results, which used to have a death rate of over 80% before antibiotics became available. Yet another variety of staphylococcal toxin causes food poisoning, and we will be returning to it in Chapter 6.

In the pre-antibiotic era, staphylococcal infections of the bones, osteomyelitis, were disabling and a long struggle to treat. As recently as 50 years ago, a treatment widely advocated involved the implantation of maggots in the putrefying tissues.

The introduction of penicillin had a miraculous effect on staphylococcal infection in the early days, but after a few years it was found that evolution of the staph population was favouring a strain which produced an enzyme, penicillinase, which made it resistant to the antibiotic. The battle against resistant staph continues to the present day.

Streptococci cause a wide variety of diseases

which were a source of great confusion for centuries after the time of Hippocrates, and it was not until bacteriologists became able to study the individual organisms at around the turn of the century that some order was brought to the proceedings. Streptococci were shown to be the organisms which caused scarlet fever, tonsillitis, otitis media, mastoiditis, meningitis, pneumonia and many other diseases including, as a late complication of throat infections, rheumatic fever. Classified into alpha, beta and gamma types according to how they destroy ('lyse') blood cells on an agar culture plate, it was found that most of the trouble was being caused by the 'beta-haemolytic' streptococci.

Like staphylococci, streptococci can be found in the majority of people in the population, favouring the throat, nose and mucous membranes of the perineum. The great majority are sensitive to penicillin and other antibiotics, which accounts for the great reductions in incidence of streptococcal diseases to have been observed in the developed world over recent years. However, these infections are related to living standards as well as to the availability of antibiotics, and streptococcal infections are still common in the developing world. Rheumatic fever, a serious complication of a streptococcal throat infection which affects the heart, has to all intents and purposes been eradicated in Britain. However, a resurgence of acute rheumatic fever has occurred in the USA: between January 1985 and June 1986, 74 cases were confirmed in Salt Lake City, and other US cities had a considerably larger number of cases reported in the mid 1980s than in previous years. It remains of world-wide significance in overcrowded communities and may possibly be increasing in incidence both in less favoured countries and in the western world.

We are constantly discovering varieties of cocci we did not know existed, and in the early days they were given names because they were associated with the diseases which were being studied. Pneumococcus, for example, got its name because it was found to be a common cause of pneumonia – but it was only later that it was found to be only one of many causes, and that practically all people – few of whom ever get pneumonia – have pneumococci living harmlessly in their throats and noses. Meningococci, similarly, were named after they were associated with meningitis – but we now know that not all meningitis is caused by meningo-

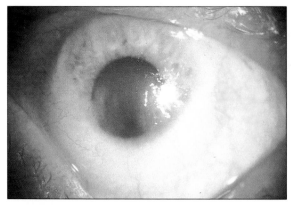

Figure 21 Trachoma of the eye caused by Chlamydia, (see page 46).

cocci, and that these bacteria are common commensals, normal inhabitants of the throats of healthy people.

It is only very rarely that the bacteria which inhabit our intestines make us ill. However, they do have close relatives which are specialised disease-producers, and these include members of the *Salmonella* and *Shigella* groups, which in their different forms cause typhoid, food poisoning, and dysentery.

Bacilli, the rod-shaped bacteria, have among their family the causative organism for anthrax, a thoroughly unpleasant disease of all mammals including man. It is rare now in Britain and other industrialised countries, but death is very likely on the even rarer occasions on which it invades parts of the body other than the skin.

Clostridia are also rod-shaped, found mostly in the soil and growing in the absence of oxygen ('anaerobic'). Members of the genus are responsible for several highly unpleasant diseases, including tetanus, gas gangrene, botulism and food poisoning.

Bacteria are classified in several ways, apart from the way they form groups. Microbiologists make use of 'Gram staining' for differentiation. During investigations into the cause of pneumonia in the late 1800s, there was great confusion when it became clear that pneumonia was not caused by one single bacterium, but it was difficult to sort out one from another. Gram, working in Berlin with dyes used for staining bacteria so that they were visible under the microscope, found that some bacteria would retain a blue dye – 'Gram positive' – whereas it could be washed out of others and replaced by a red dye – 'Gram

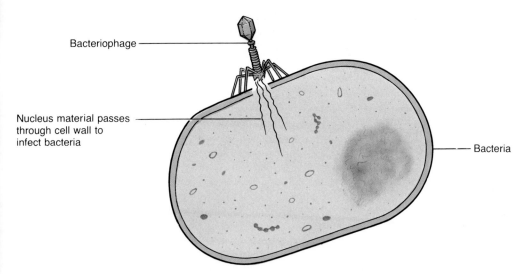

Bacteriophage

Nucleus material passes through cell wall to infect bacteria

Bacteria

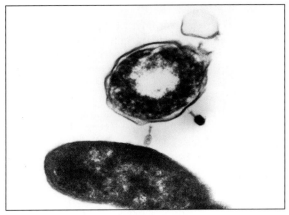

Figure 22 Some bacteria can be killed by viruses. The virus known as the bacteriophage, looking like a moon-landing vehicle, is shown here piercing the bacterial cell wall where it injects genetic material from its head into the body of the bacterium. New bacteriophages are produced and the bacterium dies, (see page 46).

(a) Diagram of a bacteriophage infecting a bacterium.

(b) Transmission electron micrograph of a T4 bacteriophage (magnification × 34,000) absorbing onto an E Coli.

negative'. This process of differentiation is still used, and bacteria in each of these two groups differ biologically and in their pathogenic effects.

Within each group (Gram positive and Gram negative) there will be bacteria which prefer to grow in the presence of oxygen (aerobes) or in the absence of oxygen (anaerobes), and a few are absolute in their preference. Hence, a particular bacterium might be described as a Gram-negative anaerobe, and all microbes of this description will have many other similarities in the causation of illness and response to antibiotics.

Within the group of organisms classed as bacteria come a few particularly small versions, and in recent years much study has been devoted to a class of organisms called *mycoplasmas*. These are particularly tiny bacteria, and can only be grown on special culture media. Interest in them arises

from the great frequency with which they are found to be associated with conditions of previously unknown origin, but the only human disease they have actually been proved to cause is a form of pneumonia.

Mycoplasmas can live out on their own, and are often found in sewage and compost as well as within living cells. But there are other tiny organisms which, like viruses, can *only* exist within living cells, and are also important causative agents of disease: the rickettsiae and the chlamydiae.

Rickettsiae are responsible for typhus, already discussed as one of the great killer diseases in times of poverty, famine and war, and for other serious fevers. They were named after Dr Howard Taylor Ricketts of Chicago, who in 1906 first transmitted the rickettsial disease Rocky Mountain spotted

'gs and monkeys, and who died of
.u City at the age of 40 years.

...iae cause the important tropical eye
.c trachoma, which is the single most impor-
.ant cause of preventable blindness in the world.
The conjunctivae of the eye become inflamed, and
secondary invasion by bacteria causes a milky
scarring of the cornea, blocking the vision.
Chlamydiae also cause lymphogranuloma vene-
reum, a tropical venereal disease which is exceeded
in prevalence only by syphilis and gonorrhoea,
and they are an important cause of 'non-specific'
urethritis.

Of more day-to-day importance in the
developed world is the now well-recognised and
important role played by the chlamydiae in the
causation of inflammatory disease of the pelvic
organs in women, a source of much illness,
hospitalisation, surgery and even infertility. The
employment of routine facilities for the diagnosis
and treatment of such infections has only very
slowly followed growing appreciation of the
importance of this organism.

Both the rickettsiae and chlamydiae can be killed
by antibiotics, which in this respect makes them
more like bacteria than viruses.

Finally, we should take notice of the bacteria
known as *spirochaetes*, which are thin-walled,
spiral and mobile. They include those which cause
syphilis, yaws and some important tropical
diseases.

Viruses

Viruses are one of the smallest and simplest of all
living things. They are the ultimate parasites,
depending absolutely on living cells – which even
include bacteria – for their continued existence.
They cannot live on their own. Partly because they
are so small, it was only a few decades ago that
their relationship to human disease could be made
clear.

Scientists working with Koch were assiduously
working through dozens of diseases which might
be due to bacteria, but in several cases they found
that the bacteria they were isolating had nothing to
do with the disease. It became clear that some other
kind of agent must be involved. The first experimental evidence that disease in vertebrates could
be caused by something such as a 'virus' (which is
Latin for poison) came in 1898 during research in

Germany on cattle foot-and-mouth disease, when
it was found that whatever was causing the disease
would pass through a porcelain filter which
blocked the passage of bacteria.

Subsequently, various preparations which had
been filtered free of any kinds of cell were over the
next 30 years used in a wide variety of important
studies. It was found, for example, that 'filterable'
agents would kill certain kinds of bacteria, and
these bacterial parasites were called 'bacteriophages'. For a time it was thought this could have
significance for treatment – indeed, their dis-
coverer, d'Herelle, suggested that by developing
suitable bacteriophages, bacterial diseases could be
eliminated – but no convincing clinical trials were
performed before antibiotics came on the scene and
this line of research was made redundant. Phages
have an important use nowadays, however,
because they are specific to various types of
bacillus. So, for example, if staphylococci are
causing problems with infection between people
('cross infection') in a hospital ward, 'phage typing'
is one of the methods that are used to sort out
which of the many types of staphylococci which
will inevitably be isolated from most of the ward
attendants' noses are in fact causing the trouble,
and this will probably narrow the search down to
one or two people.

In other pioneering work, Rous at the
Rockefeller Institute was able to show in 1911 that
a type of cancer could be passed between chickens
by way of a filtrate made from tumour material,
the first indication that some cancers might have a
viral origin.

However, progress in virus research was ham-
pered by overwhelming technical difficulties until
the 1930s, when new ways to isolate and study
viruses in the laboratory were discovered. Since
then, the pace of progress has been rapid, and
when the basic simplicity of the virus was clarified,
virology became of fundamental importance to the
emerging field of molecular biology. Two pieces of
high-technology machinery were essential to these
advances. One was the ultra-centrifuge, which
allowed viruses to be concentrated by spinning
them down, and the other was the electron microscope, which for the first time allowed them
actually to be visualised.

The other great advance was to get viruses to
replicate in the laboratory. Because they have no
independent metabolism and no life of their own
outside living cells, the early experimental work

was based on the use of small animals which could be inoculated with the preparations under study. For example, if monkeys developed poliomyelitis after a suspicious fluid was injected into their spinal cords, then it could be deduced that the fluid contained polio viruses. Similarly, ferrets – the only susceptible animals – were used to study the viruses of influenza. But the generally expensive and humanitarian difficulties of animal research are obvious, especially as it turned out that viruses were very fussy about what type of animals each one would infect. A substantial step forward came when viruses were shown to grow well on various parts of the embryo of the chicken, within the egg-shell.

In 1948 the process of 'cell culture' was perfected, and allowed very much faster and more convenient study. Human and other cells are prepared in such a way that they will grow and divide in the test tube, nourished by nutrient fluids, and the growth of viruses in such cell cultures can be seen and measured by the damage they cause to the cultured cells. The need for experimental animals finally disappeared with the development of strains of cells derived from human cancer, which have an enhanced capacity for division. These develop well in the test tube, and by planting samples from one test tube to another they can be kept in constant supply.

A virus is not an 'organism', but a very basic structure composed of a nucleic acid molecule which may be enclosed in an outer coat of protein. The nucleic acid is either of the deoxyribonucleic acid (DNA) or ribonucleic acid (RNA) type. Further classification of viruses depends on several factors, including their size and the make-up of their molecular structure, and by the structure and characteristics of their 'virions', which transmit the infections they cause.

They are all very small, with size measured in nanometres (billionths of a metre). The smallest is only just bigger than the biggest protein molecule, and the largest is about one-third of the size of the smallest staphylococcus. Only the very biggest ones, therefore, can be seen under the ordinary light microscope.

At the start of an attack by viruses, they adhere to the cell surface with the assistance of protein molecules in their membranous surface. This coating stays outside the cell, while the nucleic acid portion penetrates into the interior. New virus particles are produced within the cell, and after that process they then emerge. The infected cells may degenerate or die, or survive and continue to harbour virus particles from one cell generation to another. Inflammation may occur as a response of the tissues to substances released from the damaged cells.

Apart from enabling the virus to adhere to and penetrate the cell wall, the protein of the outer coat is antigenic and accounts for most of the immunological reactions produced by the virus. The nucleic acid part is still infectious even when separated from the protein, which shows that it carries all the genetic information necessary for developing the characteristics of the virus.

When it became possible to search for and grow viruses in the laboratory on a routine basis, it soon became clear that there were a lot more to be found than had been expected. Further, and contrary to early dark suspicions (like those which followed the isolation of the first bacteria), it was soon found that the presence of viruses was not necessarily a sign of disease. Viruses, it seemed, just like bacteria, were everywhere, mostly living with us without causing harm, even if the same viruses were well capable of causing sickness in other individuals. We are still in the early days of finding out just what does determine the course of a viral disease, and later in this chapter we examine some of the processes in the body which determine whether symptoms of sickness will result from infection.

Although we know that viruses cause a wide variety of diseases in humans, as yet we have no idea how many. As examples, the following families of virus have been shown to be responsible for clearly recognisable disease in substantial numbers of people.

Hepatitis viruses cause hepatitis A, hepatitis B, and non-A/non-B hepatitis.

Herpes viruses cause the well-known 'cold sores' of herpes simplex, and genital herpes, which is transmitted sexually. They also cause chickenpox and shingles. These are among the viruses which may cause tumours in humans, including carcinoma of the cervix; one of this group, the Epstein-Barr virus, has been associated with a type of cancer found in central Africa and with cancer of the nose and throat.

Adenoviruses occur in huge variety, causing respiratory infections and inflammation of the conjunctiva of the eye.

Papovaviruses cause warts, and may be implica-

Figure 23   Viruses can be grown in cell cultures, where human or other cells are grown in test-tubes, nourished by nutrient fluids.

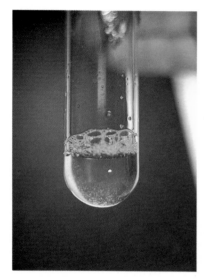

(a) Cultured cells recovered by centrifugation.

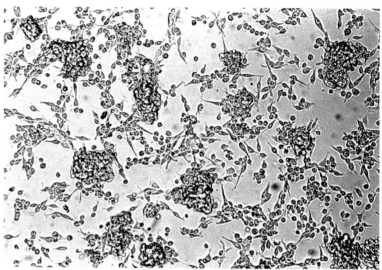

(b) Low-powered view of canine cells grown in culture.

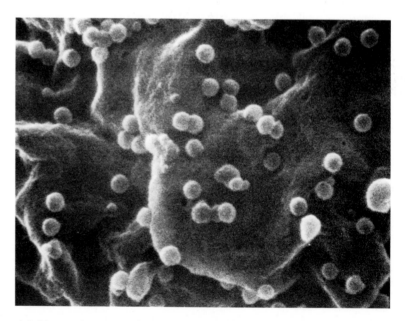

(c) Human Immunodeficiency Virus (HIV) particles shown budding from cultured lymphocytes; (magnification × 40,000).

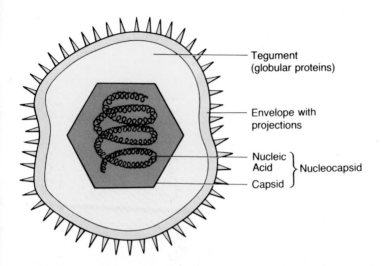

Tegument
(globular proteins)

Envelope with
projections

Nucleic
Acid } Nucleocapsid
Capsid

Figure 24 Diagram of a generalised virus. A virus is not a living organism, but a nucleic acid molecule contained within a capsule of protein. The characteristics of the infections viruses cause depend on the structure of the components of the individual virus.

Figure 25 Electron micrographs of four common viruses.
(a) Influenza; (magnification × 113,000)
(b) Hepatitis B; (magnification × 66,000)
(c) Adenovirus; (magnification × 110,000)
(d) Rotavirus; (magnification × 53,000)

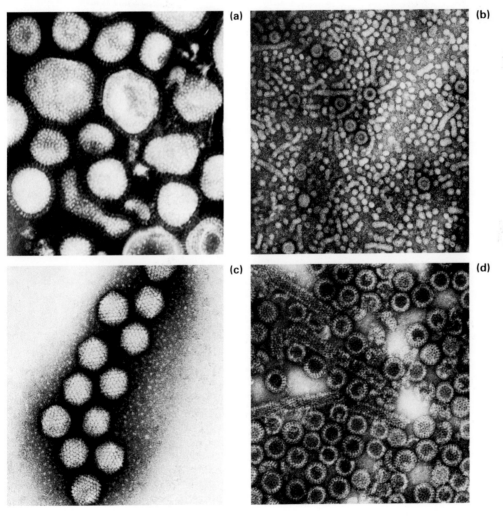

(a)

(b)

(c)

(d)

ted in the causation of carcinoma of the cervix.

Pox viruses, fortunately, are rarely seen now. The main pathogen in this group used to be small-pox, and some of the same family of diseases, such as monkeypox, still exist in the field.

Togaviruses and bunyaviruses are carried by ticks, fleas and mosquitoes; they are also therefore known as arthropod-borne, or arboviruses. Among the diseases which result are yellow fever and dengue fever.

Picornaviruses are perhaps the ones that give us the most trouble in everyday life, because the family includes the hundred or more **rhinoviruses** which are responsible for the common cold. Other respiratory infections, and poliomyelitis, are caused by viruses of this family.

Reoviruses include the **rotavirus**, comparatively recently recognised as a very important cause of gastroenteritis.

Ortho and **paramyxo viruses** are responsible for influenza, measles and mumps, and include what has comparatively recently been recognised as the major cause of respiratory tract infection in infancy, respiratory syncytial virus (RSV).

Rhabdoviruses ('bullet-shaped') include the examples which cause the much-feared rabies and the very rare Marburg fever which, previously unknown, killed several laboratory staff in Marburg who were working with a monkey from Africa.

Arenaviruses include the viruses which cause Lassa fever and a type of meningitis.

Coronaviruses are yet another family of viruses which cause infections of the upper respiratory tract.

As we have already commented, the number of diseases caused by viruses is unknown. 'New' ones keep appearing. We do not even have a good idea of the range of diseases they may be causing. For example, there are tantalising associations with a few kinds of cancer, although it has been impossible to prove cause and effect with any others. The distribution patterns of diseases such as leukaemia are more consistent with a model of spread by viral infection than with environmental cause, although the latter is the subject of greater public concern at present. It is known that some kinds of arthritis can follow virus infections. Some viruses could be associated with mental or nervous diseases; something that kills human cells in tissue culture has been identified in the cerebrospinal fluid of patients with a variety of such conditions, including schizophrenia. Two virus diseases with very long incubation periods are known to cause

degeneration of the brain which is clinically very similar to Alzheimer's disease. There are many other examples of such association, and research in fields which embrace conditions not normally recognised as 'infectious', although technically extremely difficult, will undoubtedly be active far into the future.

Protozoa

Protozoa are the smallest and simplest members of the animal family, having only one cell. They cause a range of diseases of great importance in tropical and subtropical areas, including malaria, amoebic dysentery, trypanosomiasis (sleeping sickness) and leishmaniasis. Protozoa come into the category of disease-causing organisms commonly referred to as 'parasites', and we should first perhaps clarify what this means in the context of our earlier discussion on the host-parasite relationship.

The relationship between a parasite and the host is characterised by the physical and physiological dependence of the former on the latter, as we have already described. Additional features of the relationship will be that the parasites will normally be smaller than their hosts, but exist in much bigger populations. This clearly applies in the case of the relationship between man and agents of disease such as bacteria and viruses. It also applies in the case of man's relationship with protozoa, which are one-celled animals, and metazoa, a term which embraces all animals that are not protozoa and includes the worms which are described in the next section. Rather confusingly, however, in medicine the term 'parasitology' is confined to study of protozoa and metazoa, which are members of the animal kingdom, and the diseases they cause are called 'parasitic diseases'.

Protozoa are on average much bigger than bacteria, although none of the forms that produce disease can be seen with the naked eye. They are structurally very much more advanced because they have a nucleus and a number of parts of the cell which perform many of the functions under-taken by specialised organs in more complex beings. Around the cell is the cytoplasm, which is divided into the endoplasm and the ectoplasm. The endoplasm is mainly concerned with nutritional needs, with the food being captured and taken in by the ectoplasm. Protozoa are usually capable of active movement through their use of appendages of the ectoplasm, which may include whip-like flagella or cilia, undulating wing-like membranes, or temporary extrusions known as pseudopodia.

Protozoa may be found wherever they can obtain fluid and nutrients, and stagnant ponds are well-known sources of supply for every child who has wanted to study an amoeba under the microscope. All vertebrates, including man, have abundant protozoa in their intestines, and many also live in the intestinal tracts of insects. Other protozoa live in body cavities such as the lower genital tract, mouth and lung, and many spend part of their life cycle in the blood. Intestinal protozoa frequently exist outside the body in a cystic stage, during which time active movement ceases and a firm cyst wall is secreted as a protective skin. in this form the organism is able to survive under most reasonably favourable environmental circumstances until it is taken in by a new host with water or food.

A feature of the life of a typical protozoan is its cycle of stages, which is particularly complex in the case of those which are responsible for blood infections, such as malaria. In such cases, the parasite depends for part of its existence on a blood-sucking arthropod, such as a mosquito or a sand-fly. Protozoa reproduce either asexually, by simple division of the cell, or sexually by division of the cell after fertilisation, and frequently one form of reproduction takes place in man while the other occurs in the arthropod intermediary.

One of the few protozoal diseases common in Britain is really a zoonosis, a disease of cats: toxoplasmosis, caused by *Toxoplasma gondii*. Toxoplasma infection is acquired by ingestion of the organism, either as a result of close contact with cats or from eating the raw or lightly-cooked meat of animals which can be intermediate hosts for the organism, such as cattle or pigs. The organism then finds its way all over the body and causes a generalised, vague, feverish illness which is rarely severe. However, if a pregnant woman is infected during the first three months of pregnancy the foetus can become infected, which may result in congenital disease or malformation, stillbirth or abortion. Cats should be kept away from food, especially when the cook is pregnant. Severe disease can result in infected individuals whose immune system is deficient, such as those with AIDS.

Of the protozoal diseases of the intestine, by far the most common is amoebiasis, characterised by amoebic dysentery. The infection is caused by an amoeba called *Entamoeba histolytica*, and the result is both acute and chronic diarrhoea. The more serious forms of this disease are a major problem in parts of Africa, South-East Asia, China, and Latin America, especially Mexico. When inadequate sanitary conditions and the presence of particularly virulent forms of the amoeba combine, a high incidence of the infection and its complications will be sustained. In Mexico City some 15% of cases of acute diarrhoea in children requiring hospitalisation have been found to be associated with *E. histolytica*.

The amoeba in question is a very unspecialised animal, similar to the one frequently found swimming in ponds, but it has developed the capacity to digest particles of food in the intestine by secreting an enzyme and then engulfing the breakdown products. During a disease caused by the more virulent variety, the amoeba invades the lining of the intestine in order to draw its nourishment in the same manner from red blood cells and tissues of the intestinal wall. This causes ulceration and bleeding, with the symptoms of dysentery: persistent diarrhoea with blood and slimy mucus in the stools. A serious complication is that the amoebae may enter the blood and spread to the liver, where they can multiply and cause an abscess.

The amoebae are excreted in the faeces as cysts, and after being swallowed in contaminated food or water by the next host, again take up their amoebic form.

These amoebae show a wide difference in virulence, and many people who live and travel in the tropics harbour them in their bowel without suffering any symptoms. There are many possible reasons for this, in addition to differences in virulence between strains of amoebae: resistance to disease, for example, may depend on the general state of health and nutrition, and it may be easier for an amoeba to invade the wall of an intestine which is already damaged by another infection. On the other hand, long association between host and parasite may lead to a working relationship, as in other cases of infection.

Dysentery sometimes flares up after travellers have returned from the tropics, and of course any individual excreting cysts in the faeces, whether frankly ill at the time or not, is a potential threat to others. Effective drug treatment is now available.

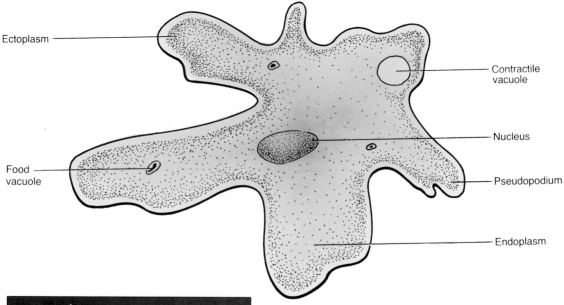

Ectoplasm

Contractile vacuole

Nucleus

Food vacuole

Pseudopodium

Endoplasm

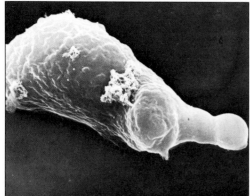

Figure 26 Protozoa are the smallest members of the animal world, and they have all the structures of an organism, including basic feeding and excretory systems.

(a) Diagram to show structure of amoeba.

(b) Scanning electron micrograph of Entamoeba Histolytica, which causes dysentery (magnification × 2,000).

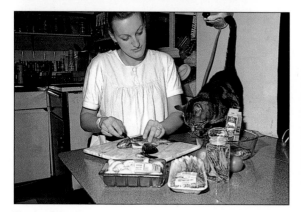

Figure 27 Toxoplasmosis is a protozoal disease which is carried by cats and can be transmitted to humans. The infection can cause deformation and other damage to the human foetus.

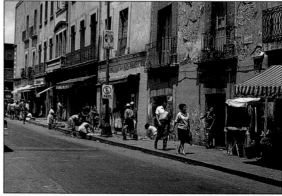

Figure 28 A street in Mexico City. Amoebae can colonise the human intestinal tract and cause amoebic dysentery, common in crowded cities with inadequate public water and sewerage facilities.

Figure 29 The complex life cycle of the malaria parasite. Regular episodes of fever occur when immense batches of merozoites are released into the blood.

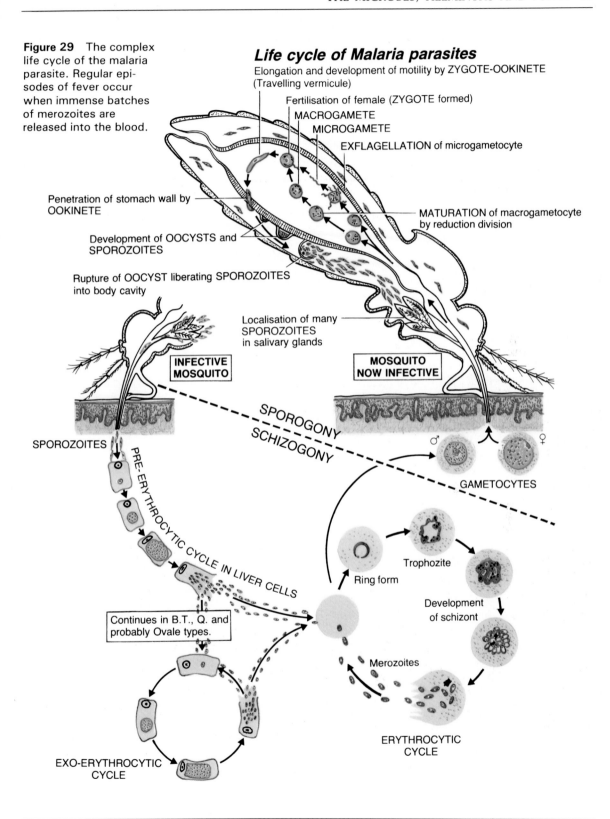

Life cycle of Malaria parasites

Elongation and development of motility by ZYGOTE-OOKINETE (Travelling vermicule)

Fertilisation of female (ZYGOTE formed)

MACROGAMETE

MICROGAMETE

EXFLAGELLATION of microgametocyte

Penetration of stomach wall by OOKINETE

MATURATION of macrogametocyte by reduction division

Development of OOCYSTS and SPOROZOITES

Rupture of OOCYST liberating SPOROZOITES into body cavity

Localisation of many SPOROZOITES in salivary glands

INFECTIVE MOSQUITO

MOSQUITO NOW INFECTIVE

SPOROZOITES

SPOROGONY

SCHIZOGONY

PRE-ERYTHROCYTIC CYCLE IN LIVER CELLS

♂ ♀

GAMETOCYTES

Ring form

Trophozite

Development of schizont

Merozoites

Continues in B.T., Q. and probably Ovale types.

EXO-ERYTHROCYTIC CYCLE

ERYTHROCYTIC CYCLE

Another cause of intestinal parasitic infection is the flagellate *Giardia lamblia* (*G. intestinalis*), which may be encountered anywhere in the world, and especially Africa, Asia and Latin America. It is one of the most common causes of diarrhoea among children in the developing countries. In Britain and the United States it is the most commonly reported intestinal parasitic infection of man, and a common cause of 'travellers' diarrhoea'; in 1983, in the USA, *Giardia* was identified as the cause of 68% of waterborne outbreaks of diarrhoea in which the cause was known. A wide variety of stomach symptoms can follow infection and, with or without symptoms, individuals can excrete cysts for months.

A very much more complicated life cycle is a feature of the protozoa which are parasites of the blood, among which malarial protozoa are perhaps the most important: Sir Macfarlane Burnet stated that of all the infectious diseases there was no doubt that malaria caused the greatest harm to the greatest number. Thousands of people seen by doctors each year in Britain are suffering from malaria, although they will have contracted it somewhere else. Since 1970 there has been a worldwide resurgence of this disease, with a peak in 1976 and then a decline, so that by 1982 the number of reported cases was similar to that reported in 1974. In general, there has been very little progress in control in many countries; indeed, there has been a deterioration in some areas. The actual number of new cases each year in the world may be in the order of 92 million. We will be discussing many aspects of this disease in various parts of this book; here, we are concerned only with the characteristics of the infecting organism.

There are four species of the micro-organism *Plasmodium* which infect man, of which three are responsible for nearly all cases of human disease. They all have a similar life cycle, part of which takes place in man and part in the disease vectors, several species of mosquito of the genus *Anopheles*.

We pick up the cycle as the mosquito bites (or, more accurately, stabs) its victim in order to suck blood. To stop the blood clotting, it injects an anticoagulant from its salivary glands, and minute forms of the parasite ('sporozoites') are injected with it into the blood capillaries. Within an hour of entering the circulation the sporozoites enter the liver and penetrate the liver cells, where they enlarge and multiply. After between five and

fifteen days, depending on the type, the cells rupture and release thousands of what are then known as 'merozoites' into the bloodstream, where some of them become attached to and then enter red blood cells. Here, they grow into 'trophozoites' (in which form they are visible under the microscope) and then 'schizonts'. These divide rapidly, and when finally the remnants of the red blood cell break down, dozens of new merozoites are liberated into the blood, where they latch on to a new batch of red blood cells.

Fever occurs when the merozoites are released, which explains its cyclic nature: it takes two to three days for parasites in the newly infected blood cells to build up their numbers and burst out again. The number and severity of the attacks of fever vary according to the virulence of the strain of malaria, the general health of the infected individual, the treatment he receives and so on. If no treatment is offered, white blood cells and antibodies gradually destroy the parasites, but small numbers of them may remain in the bloodstream, liver and other organs for years afterward.

Several days after the first parasites become detectable in the blood, new forms of the trophozoite appear. These are sexually differentiated 'gametocytes', and it is they that infect any mosquito of the right species that sucks the blood of the person at that stage. In the intestine of the mosquito the male and female forms unite, producing up to a thousand new sporozoites at a time, and some of these bore their way through to the ducts of the mosquito's salivary glands, ready to be injected into a new victim. The duration of this mosquito part of the parasite life cycle is between 10 and 20 days, which is of obvious importance to the epidemiology and control of malaria, since transmission can only occur if the mosquito lives long enough after biting someone to pass on the infection to a new victim.

Trypanosomes are the protozoa which cause sleeping sickness (trypanosomiasis), a disease which has devastated large areas of central Africa. It was originally spread with the animals and humans involved in the slave trade; in present times, outbreaks are likely to occur when social systems are broken down by disruptions such as war and famine, and people move into endemic areas. In east Africa it is primarily a disease of animals, and is transmitted from them to man by the bite of the tsetse fly; in west Africa, a slightly different form is transmitted from person to person in the same way. Many wild animals act as a reservoir for trypanosomes without suffering, but infection of domestic animals (including cattle and horses) can cause death, a matter of great economic concern.

The tsetse fly cycle begins when the insect sucks infected blood, and the protozoa multiply in the insect's gut. After about two to four weeks the trypanosomes reach the salivary glands, from which they are injected, and the fly remains capable of spreading the infection for at least three months.

In Central and South America, millions of people are affected by another type of trypanosome, transmitted by a large bug which comes out at night to bite, called *Triatoma*, or – locally – the 'kissing bug'. In *The Voyage of the Beagle* Charles Darwin vividly describes being bitten by these bugs, and it has been suggested that it was the South American form of trypanosomiasis, called Chagas' disease, that was responsible for the chronic illness which has puzzled his biographers. The bug does not inject the parasite but deposits it in faeces, which are then introduced into the bloodstream when the victim scratches. Unlike African trypanosomes they do not multiply in the blood but become localised in various organs, where they can cause a diffuse variety of symptoms, hard to diagnose.

The leishmaniases are a group of conditions of importance to public health which are spreading in distribution and increasing in incidence. Protozoa of the genus *Leishmania* form a large group, and they infect a wide range of vertebrates including man. The range of diseases they cause is large, too, although they fall into three main categories: cutaneous leishmaniasis, which forms a persistent ulcerating sore (known as 'Oriental sore' and many other popular local names, this lesion can leave a disfiguring scar); mucocutaneous leishmaniasis, which can eat away in a horribly mutilating manner the linings of the nose, throat and mouth; and visceral leishmaniasis, a disease which affects many organs of the body, especially the liver and spleen. Visceral leishmaniasis is also known as kala azar, or 'black sickness', because of the darkening of the skin it causes. Around the turn of the century, kala azar was recognised as one of the scourges of South-East Asia, and it is known to have existed for centuries in India, China, Africa and the Mediterranean basin. If untreated, it is often fatal, but effective drugs are now available.

Today, both the skin and visceral forms of the disease are distributed in South America, Africa, the Mediterranean, the Near East and India.

The life histories of the responsible protozoa all include various types of sandfly, which bite and suck blood at dusk, dawn and in the night. The organisms multiply over the next two or three weeks in the stomach of the sandfly to produce large numbers of freely mobile forms, and some are regurgitated – and thus infect the new victim – before fresh blood is ingested. Dogs and rodents, especially in big cities, can act as reservoirs.

HELMINTHS

There are numerous multicelled animals (metazoa) which are parasites on man and commonly known as worms. These are much larger than the one-celled creatures we have described so far, and can vary in length from about 1 mm to over 6 metres. Many millions of people in the world suffer illness because of worm infestation, but most of the serious cases seen in Britain have been imported from tropical and subtropical countries.

Helminths have a complicated structure and life cycle with sexually reproducing adult stages and a sequence of development passing from the egg or embryo, through various larval or nymphal stages to the sexually mature adult. An infected human may be host to the larval stages of some parasites and the adult stages of other different ones, and a host is commonly infected by both the larval and adult stages of one species. However, part of the life cycle of an individual helminth will almost always be completed outside the host, so that unless reinfection occurs – which, in the areas where helminthic infection is prevalent, is always likely – the number of parasites does not increase. In general, whereas protozoa multiply within their hosts, metazoa build up their numbers by accumulation.

The life cycles of the helminthic parasites are very long in comparison with those of the protozoa, some worms taking 18 months or so to reach maturity and then leading a long life, up to 25 years in the case of a beef tapeworm or even 40 years for a liver fluke. This means that genetic change takes place at a very slow pace, and the worms tend not, therefore, to become resistant to the generally effective drugs used to kill them.

Figure 30 Macrophotograph of mosquito *Anopheles balabacensis* feeding on human blood; (magnification × 11).

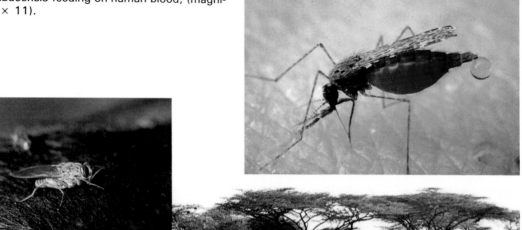

Figure 31 Trypanosomiasis is primarily a disease of animals, such as pigs, carried by the tsetse fly and transmitted to man by its bite.

Figure 32 Leishmaniasis is an important protozoal disease of man spread by the sandfly. It causes a range of diseases: the two main forms are cutaneous ('Oriental sores') and visceral affecting many organs of the body.

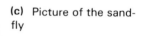

(a) 'Oriental sore' — lesion caused by cutaneous Leishmaniasis

(b) Spleen cell showing Leishmaniasis organism

(c) Picture of the sandfly

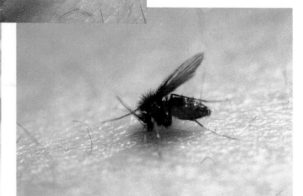

Figure 33 The life-cycle of the Ascaris roundworm is a typical example of parasitism of man by a member of the worm family.

Ascaris lumbricoides (The round worm)

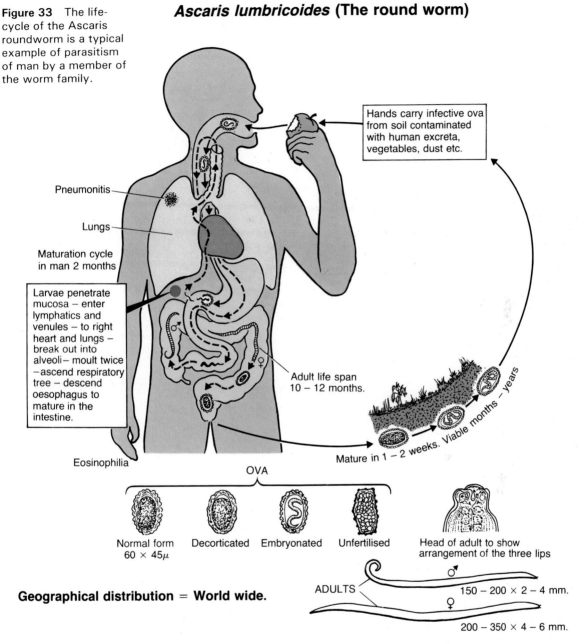

Hands carry infective ova from soil contaminated with human excreta, vegetables, dust etc.

Pneumonitis

Lungs

Maturation cycle in man 2 months

Larvae penetrate mucosa – enter lymphatics and venules – to right heart and lungs – break out into alveoli – moult twice – ascend respiratory tree – descend oesophagus to mature in the intestine.

Adult life span 10 – 12 months.

Mature in 1 – 2 weeks. Viable months – years

Eosinophilia

OVA

Normal form 60 × 45μ

Decorticated

Embryonated

Unfertilised

Head of adult to show arrangement of the three lips

Geographical distribution = World wide.

ADULTS

♂   150 – 200 × 2 – 4 mm.

♀   200 – 350 × 4 – 6 mm.

PATHOLOGY

LARVAE Allergy, eosinophilia and pneumonitis. Occasionally larvae in other organs with local inflammation and necrosis.

ADULTS Obstruction of intestine, bile ducts and trachea have been reported.

LABORATORY DIAGNOSIS

Recovery of ova from faeces. Rarely embryos may be found in sputum.

They are found in all parts of the world as parasites of virtually all vertebrates, in which most of them spend most of their lives. A few helminths spend at least part of their life cycle in the free state, usually in soil or water.

Helminths are divided into two main groups: roundworms (*nematodes*), which cause diseases such as ascariasis, ancylostomiasis (caused by hookworms), filariasis, trichuriasis, and trichinosis; and flatworms (*trematodes* and *cestodes*). The trematodes are also known as flukes, and among the important diseases they cause is schistosomiasis. Cestodes include the fish tapeworm, the beef and pork tapeworms, and hydatid disease.

Roundworms infest a high proportion of the world's total population, with estimates (necessarily rough) being in the order of 1000 million cases of ascariasis, 900 million for hookworms, and 500 million for trichinosis. Many of these people, of course, are infected with more than one type of worm at a time.

The roundworms of *Ascaris lumbricoides* are 15 to 45 cm in length and 2 to 6 mm in diameter. They produce prodigious numbers of eggs, which may remain viable in the soil for many months, and reach man through contamination of food, often vegetables. The eggs hatch in the small intestine and the larvae penetrate the wall of the gut to get into the bloodstream. They migrate to the lungs, from where they are coughed up and swallowed back into the intestine, where they then grow into maturity. Infections involving only a few worms cause little or no problem, but heavy infections deprive the host of his food (which may in any case be limited in supply), and cause intestinal discomfort and possibly blockage of the gut or bile ducts. They certainly upset the nutritional status of children.

Ascariasis abounds in many areas of the world where the weather is warm and human faeces are disposed of carelessly or used as fertilizer. The infestation affects about one-third of the population of Africa, with a higher incidence in children than adults, and wide differences between locations. In Brazil, the incidence in various regions has been measured at between 27 and 98%. Over half the children admitted to the Rangoon Children's Hospital with acute abdominal problems have been found to be suffering from ascariasis. Drug treatment is effective when it can be administered.

The bloodsucking nematodes *Ancylostoma* and *Necator* are known as *hookworms* because of the way the adults feed. About one centimetre long, they attach themselves to the wall of the small intestine with their specially adapted, toothlike mouth parts and suck blood from the capillary blood vessels. Eggs from the female worms are passed in the faeces, and the embryos within the eggs develop rapidly in warm and moist conditions. The larvae hatch in 5–10 days, and can survive for up to a month in the tropics. Infection occurs when the larvae penetrate the skin (which can be intact), usually of the feet. In the blood they migrate to the lungs, where they may cause a cough, and then back down the oesophagus to the gut. Hookworm infection causes blood loss and depletion of the body's stores of iron, leading to iron-deficiency anaemia. Each worm can cause the daily loss into the intestine of 0.14–0.26 ml of blood, and because several hundred hookworms may all be feeding at the same time the blood loss can easily cause anaemia even when the dietary iron intake is high, let alone when it is not.

The larvae of hookworms that normally parasitise cats and dogs may penetrate human skin but do not move into the blood, instead wandering underneath the skin surface and causing very itchy red streaks. They are commonly picked up by people using beaches in the Americas, Africa and Asia which have been befouled by dogs.

Considering its worldwide distribution and high prevalence, trichuriasis, caused by the nematode *Trichuris trichiura*, has been neglected more than the other parasitic diseases of the intestine. The illness associated with the infestation is due to the worm's unique mode of attachment to the intestinal wall, most commonly in the large bowel. Each worm is about 50 mm long, with a thin front part which it burrows into the flesh and uses to feed on the tissues of the intestine. This may cause ulceration of the intestinal lining, and not surprisingly is associated with chronic nutritional disorder and diarrhoea. Each female worm pours out 2,000–14,000 eggs a day, which are swallowed by new hosts after the usual passage over the ground.

Quite common in the tropical areas of the world is filariasis, a condition which is caused by several varieties of a long and thread-like nematode worm. They live for a long time in the body, but unless present in very high numbers cause few if any ill effects. Filariasis was the first human disease in which the role of an intermediate was proved; that it is transmitted by the bite of a mosquito was discovered by Patrick Manson in 1877 while practising medicine in colonial China. Manson was a Scottish doctor later to become a famous leader in the field of tropical medicine.

The worms live in the lymph glands and vessels, and a very small proportion of people living in areas with heavy infestation develop an incapacitating swelling of the legs and arms called elephantiasis. Filariasis was once very common in the Pacific islands, and thousands of soldiers became infected in the Pacific during the second world war.

A rather rare form of filariasis produces a disease, onchocerciasis, which is transmitted from man to man by the bite of black flies of the family *Simuliidae*. The worms group in nodules under the skin, and can invade the eye to cause visual difficulty or even blindness, common in central Africa.

Trichinosis, caused by the worm *Trichinella spiralis*, is primarily a disease of pigs, and man becomes infected by eating inadequately cooked pork which has the cyst form in the muscle tissue. It is now quite rare in the developed world, but it has an interesting history. Several outbreaks of the disease occurred in Germany during the latter part of the nineteenth century, and Germany and some other European countries banned the importation of pork from the United States. To the States, however, this was a massively important export, and the first report of the brand new United States Public Health Service was on trichinosis; a draft of this report exonerated the producers and exports resumed. Trichinella are also found in polar bears, and one account has it that a party of Scandinavian scientists who travelled to the Arctic by balloon died after eating infected polar bear. Their frozen remains still contained trichinella larvae when they were discovered 33 years later.

In Britain, probably the commonest roundworm infestation is by the threadworm, or pinworm, *Enterobius vermicularis*, which undergoes its complete life cycle in man. Eggs are swallowed, the worms develop in the gut, and the females emerge at night to deposit their eggs on the skin around the anus. This process itches, the eggs are transferred to the fingers, and thus into the mouth of the same individual or someone else. Good personal hygiene breaks the cycle of infection, and effective drug treatment is available.

The most important disease caused by *trematodes*, or flatworms, is schistosomiasis (Fig. 38). It is also known as bilharzia, after Dr Theodor Bilharz, who discovered in 1851 the worms that cause the disease. Schistosomiasis is a disease

which examination of mummies has shown has existed along the Nile Valley since ancient times. Before the first world war Lord Kitchener, then High Commissioner of Egypt, recognised the serious nature of the disease in that country and stimulated a series of studies by university and army groups over the next few years which worked out the complicated life cycle of the schistosomes.

Schistosomes are also known as blood flukes. Man is the definitive host for the worms, male and female pairs of which become attached to the walls of large veins of the lower intestine and bladder. They are from 10 to 20 mm in length. In large numbers the eggs pass from the body in the urine or faeces, and the successful ones will find themselves in fresh water which is used for bathing and drinking. Larvae from the hatched eggs swim freely until they encounter certain types of snail, which are necessary as intermediate hosts for the parasite. After some three weeks of development in the soft tissue of the snail, what are then known as cercariae emerge, and these then actively seek out people who swim in the contaminated water or drink it. The cercariae digest their way through the skin or mucous membrane and into the bloodstream, becoming sexually differentiated in the blood vessels of the liver and from there back down – against the bloodstream – to the veins of the lower intestine and bladder. A single infected person who is passing eggs daily can infect a whole river if there are plenty of appropriate snails in the water, and thus passage of the infection is almost inevitable.

Illness results from chronic inflammation of the intestinal and bladder walls, and is associated with weakness, anaemia and longstanding debilitation. Sometimes the larvae die in the skin, causing a rash and intense irritation which is known as 'swimmers' itch', a not uncommon affliction of travellers who cannot resist a dip in cooling water.

Schistosomiasis is distributed widely throughout the tropical and subtropical areas of the world, many of which are poor and undeveloped. Ironically, the disease is associated with economic developments which are intended to break the cycle of poverty and disease, such as the building of dams and water supply systems for drinking and irrigation. These new bodies of water are all that the intermediary snail requires in order to move into pristine hunting grounds.

Like other examples of the major illnesses, schistosomiasis has played its part in the affairs of

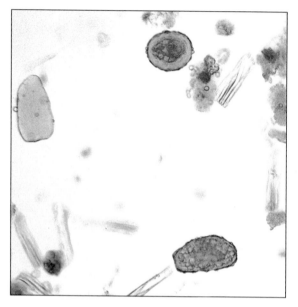

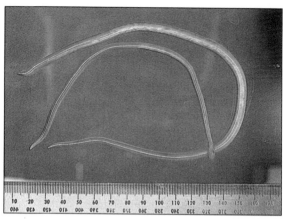

Figure 34 *Ascaris Lumbricoides* roundworm infection is endemic in tropical countries, especially in rural areas where poor hygiene and inadequate sanitation facilities exist.

(a) Egg of roundworm

(b) Adult round worms

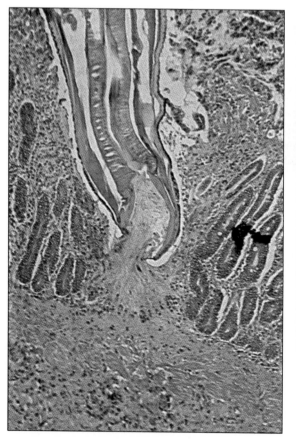

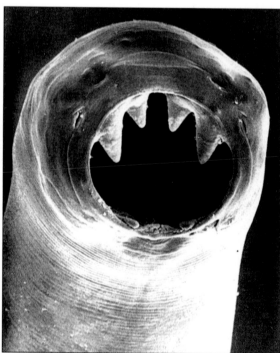

Figure 35 Hookworm nematode.

(a) *Ancylostoma*.

(b) Cross section of hookworm in the small intestine

Figure 36

The Hookworms

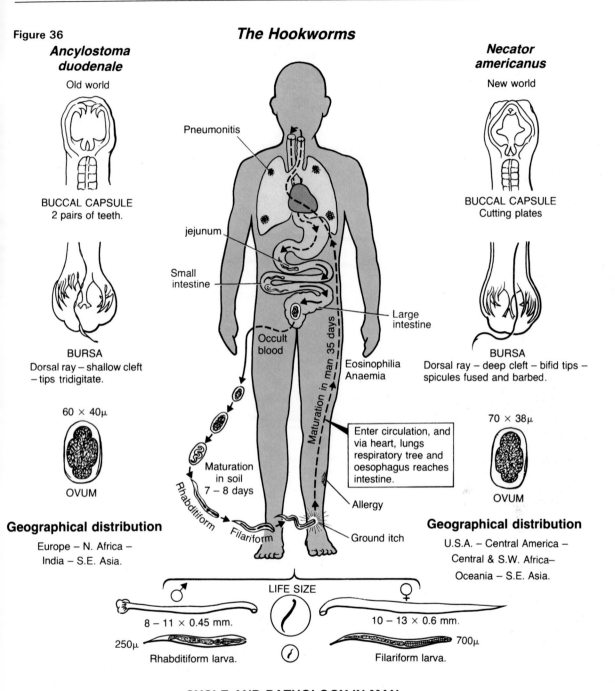

Ancylostoma duodenale

Old world

BUCCAL CAPSULE
2 pairs of teeth.

BURSA
Dorsal ray – shallow cleft
– tips tridigitate.

$60 \times 40\mu$

OVUM

Geographical distribution

Europe – N. Africa –
India – S.E. Asia.

Necator americanus

New world

BUCCAL CAPSULE
Cutting plates

BURSA
Dorsal ray – deep cleft – bifid tips –
spicules fused and barbed.

$70 \times 38\mu$

OVUM

Geographical distribution

U.S.A. – Central America –
Central & S.W. Africa–
Oceania – S.E. Asia.

Pneumonitis

jejunum

Small intestine

Large intestine

Occult blood

Maturation in man 35 days

Eosinophilia
Anaemia

Enter circulation, and via heart, lungs respiratory tree and oesophagus reaches intestine.

Allergy

Ground itch

Maturation in soil 7 – 8 days

Rhabditiform

Filariform

LIFE SIZE

♂ 8 – 11 × 0.45 mm.

♀ 10 – 13 × 0.6 mm.

250μ Rhabditiform larva.

700μ Filariform larva.

CYCLE AND PATHOLOGY IN MAN

1. Infection .... General allergic reactions – ground itch – cutaneous larva migrans in non-human ancylostomes.
2. Migration .... Lung involvement – localised pneumonitis – eosinophilia – allergy.
3. Localisation ... In jejunum – ingestion of blood by parasites – occult bleeding from intestinal mucosa – anaemia (and sequalae).

LABORATORY DIAGNOSIS

Ova in stools.

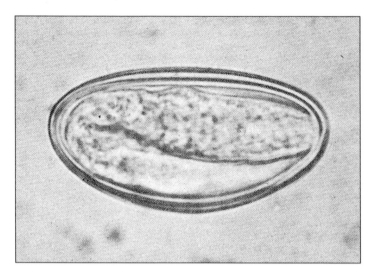

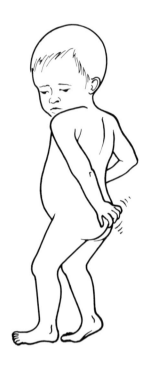

Figure 37   One of the commonest worm infestations in Britain is caused by the thread worm, (*enterobius vermicularis*).

The eggs of the worm are carried from the anus on the fingers and spread can be controlled by good personal hygiene and the use of specified drugs.

mankind, changing in some way the course of history. After American troops invaded Leyte in the Philippines in 1944, many of them became infected with the parasite. By 1946 hundreds of cases had been diagnosed, with subsequent withdrawal from the area resulting in recovery. Another story from the time of the second world war is that Mao Tse Tung's communist army was trained in the canals of China for an invasion of Taiwan, but 30–50 thousand men became incapacitated and the invasion had to be called off.

Cestodes, or tapeworms, in the adult stage are segmented flatworms, made up of a head, neck, and a series of segments (Fig. 39). The head is adapted for attachment to the wall of the intestine; the whole parasite may reach a length of over six metres. The eggs are discharged in the faeces. Man is the definitive host for both beef and pork tapeworms.

The disease is spread by the presence of human faeces where cattle and pigs feed. The next stage of the cycle depends on the particular type of worm. In the case of the beef tapeworm, *Taenia saginata*, the faeces are taken up by cattle grazing in contaminated pastures, and the larvae reach the flesh of the animal via the bloodstream. Man is infected by eating raw or undercooked beef, but infection

rarely causes severe clinical problems. Much more serious is infection with the pork tapeworm, where the main difference in the life cycle is that if man ingests the eggs directly, the larvae get into the blood and are dispersed throughout the body. In any location, then, they can become encysted, a condition known as cysticercosis. Cysts in the brain or other parts of the central nervous system represent a serious threat, being capable of causing epilepsy, mental degeneration and death. Like most helminthic infestation, the disease can now be effectively treated with drugs.

The fish tapeworm is rarely serious, but can cause anaemia. It is acquired by eating raw fish.

Finally, a tapeworm which occasionally affects man is one that lives in the intestines of dogs, *Echinococcus granulosus*. Dogs become infected when they eat the internal organs of sheep or other animals that contain larvae in cystic form. The eggs of the mature parasite are passed in dogs' faeces, and humans are usually infected by stroking the animals. Within humans larval cysts, generally known as hydatid cysts, form in the liver, lungs and other organs. They act like cancerous tumours, growing sometimes very large and needing surgical excision.

It is a rare condition in most countries, but can

be found wherever sheep are farmed and the dogs are fed on sheep offal. In many places, including Iceland, New Zealand and Tasmania, intense educational efforts directed at farmers have shown how the transmission cycle can be blocked, and have been very successful.

FUNGI

There are at least 100,000 species of fungi, but only about 50 of them affect man as potential pathogens. These belong in the class 'fungi imperfecti', and occur in four main groups.

- *Filamentous fungi* grow in long thin filaments, or 'hyphae', intertwining to form a 'mycelium'. They reproduce by spores.
- *Yeasts* are round or oval single cells, reproducing by budding from the parent cell.
- *Yeast-like fungi* are also round and oval cells reproducing by budding, but they can also form filaments.
- *Dimorphic fungi* grow as yeast in the body, but in the environment or when being cultured artificially they also form mycelia.

Fungi can cause many diseases, but the study of the 'mycoses' started as a branch of dermatology because the first human fungal diseases to be identified were all conditions of the skin. Mycology also developed as a science through the work of botanists and agriculturalists. It was a fungus disease of potatoes which wrecked the Irish crop in the mid-nineteenth century, leading to great suffering and thousands of deaths from famine, and this was one of many examples of fungal disease causing harm indirectly to humans through their effects on foodstuffs. But medical mycology was not a subject of very intense study until the 1930s and '40s.

The diseases of man caused by fungi can be divided into those that affect the skin, and those that affect the body as a whole.

Superficial fungal infections of the skin are caused by what are known as dermatophytes, fungi which invade only 'dead' tissues of the skin or its appendages, such as the corneal layer of the skin, the nails, hair and so on. A well-known word which is virtually synonymous with dermato-

phytosis is *tinea*. The genera most commonly involved are: *Microsporum*, which gives rise to tinea, or 'ringworm', mostly of the scalp; *Trichophyton*, tinea of the body and nails, and 'athlete's foot'; and *Epidermophyton*. These infections are widely known and recognised; transmission is direct from skin to skin or indirect via combs and clippers or the backs of seats. One species of *Microsporum* is common on cats and dogs and is often picked up by children.

A mycosis which affects not only the skin but also the mucous membranes is known as candidiasis, and is caused mostly by *Candida albicans*. Humans are the only reservoir of *Candida*. It is a normal commensal of about one-third of the population; the vagina commonly harbours the organism in manageable quantities, balanced by the remainder of the normal vaginal flora. It occasionally gives rise to local inflammation of the vagina ('vaginal candidiasis'), especially before puberty and after the menopause, when the acidity of the vaginal fluids is such as to encourage its growth. The symptoms include a discharge and an unrelenting, troublesome itch.

Infection of the mouth is often called thrush, a condition which can be severe in infants. Transmission of candidiasis is by direct contact or through the faeces, but the simple existence of this commensal in a given site does not mean that it has necessarily been transferred there by contact.

Candidiasis can sometimes follow a course of antibiotics for some unrelated infection such as tonsillitis, during which other commensals (including those in the vagina) are destroyed fortuitously and candida, unopposed, flourish unrestrained.

Among the factors which predispose to candidiasis – which may be the reasons for which medical attention is first sought – are general debilitation, diabetes, and chemotherapy, radiotherapy or other reasons for deficiencies in the body's immune system. Especially in such people, *Candida* can invade the bloodstream and infect the internal body systems; the resulting illness, 'systemic' candidiasis, is often a very serious one. In hospitals, systemic candidiasis may be associated with injections or the use of catheters.

In tropical and subtropical areas, especially where people go barefoot, a variety of fungi may become implanted under the skin by thorns, and give rise to a chronic, suppurating swelling called a mycetoma. Less serious, another fungal disease

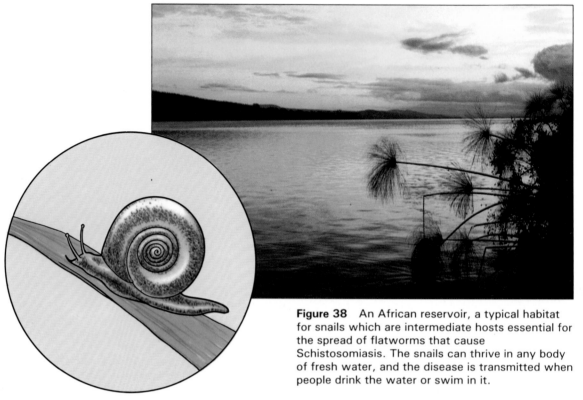

Figure 38   An African reservoir, a typical habitat for snails which are intermediate hosts essential for the spread of flatworms that cause Schistosomiasis. The snails can thrive in any body of fresh water, and the disease is transmitted when people drink the water or swim in it.

planted under the skin by natural injection of this kind is caused by the dimorphic fungus *Sporothrix schenckii*; reported from all over the world, it appears to be an occupational hazard of gardeners and horticulturalists.

The systemic, or deep mycoses are caused by fungi which are usually not pathogenic unless they enter a host whose ability to resist infection is compromised by one of the predisposing factors mentioned above; that is, the fungi are 'opportunistic'. In such patients the infection is usually serious and difficult to treat; opportunistic fungal infections are a feature of the clinical course of the acquired immune deficiency syndrome (AIDS).

Those that are primary, rather than opportunistic, infections tend to occur in typical geographical locations, so that they may be well known in a particular area but present great diagnostic difficulty if travellers come home with symptoms which have developed after a period of time. Virtually all primary deep mycoses have a chronic course, without intense or dramatic symptoms. Diagnosis is usually only possible by isolating the fungus, but because many of them are

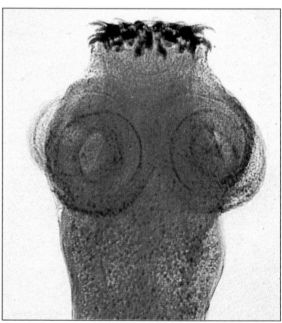

Figure 39   The head of the tapeworm has hooks and suckers to enable it to attach to the host's intestine. (see page 54)

commensals even that may be difficult unless actual invasion of the tissues can be demonstrated. A few of the more important systemic mycoses are as follows.

Histoplasmosis is caused by *Histoplasma capsulatum*. It was first described in Panama in 1906, but was confused with tuberculosis; it was later found to be widely distributed throughout all continents, especially the United States, but it rarely causes clinical disease. The spores which spread the fungus are found in the dust of old chicken coops and the caves which are home to bats.

Another systemic mycosis found in the dry areas of the Americas is coccidioidomycosis, which, like histoplasmosis, can cause respiratory complaints or any other vague symptoms. It is caused by the dimorphic fungus *Coccidioides immitis*. Confined to certain localities, it gets local names like 'valley fever' in the San Joaquin Valley.

A yeast causes cryptococcosis, or torulosis, which may be found sporadically anywhere in the world. Blastomycosis, a rare but related disease, is found in the Americas and Middle East. Aspergillosis and mucormycosis are two more of the more commonly encountered, but still rare in fit people, systemic mycoses.

Aspergillus flavus, however, has another claim to fame: it produces a particularly unpleasant 'mycotoxin'. Fungi not only invade the tissues but also, like some bacteria, can produce toxins. Growing on certain foods *A. flavus* produces aflatoxin, which has been shown to be highly carcinogenic in experimental animals as well as causing other diseases in animals and fish. It has long been recognised that fungi can be poisonous to man and animals. Contamination of rye by the fungus *Claviceps purpura* causes ergotism, which has occurred in severe epidemic form on many occasions over the centuries. St Anthony's fire, as it was known in the Middle Ages, caused intense pain and sometimes gangrene of the extremities. However, it was not until comparatively recently that renewed interest in the mycotoxins was caused by their devastating effects on reared animals. A spectacular case was the death of 100,000 young turkeys in England in 1960 after eating peanuts contaminated by *A. flavus*, and suddenly the aflatoxins became a popular subject for scientific study. The problem for humans is in the developing countries, where mycotoxin contamination of grain poses a hazard to those who are in a poor technological position to counter it.

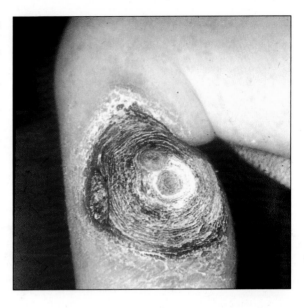

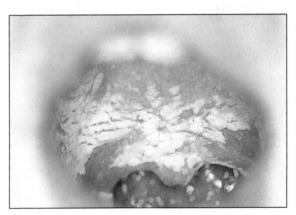

Figure 40 Fungal infections can affect skin, mucous membranes or internal organs of the body and often follows disturbance in the immune system

(a) Aspergilla can cause invasive infections of the skin and internal organs

(b) Candida Albicans (thrush) causes an infection of the mouth

5

Invasion and Response

PATHOGENICITY

The great majority of micro-organisms living on and in the body are normally harmless. Commensal flora are to be found on the skin and mucous membranes and in the intestinal tract. Under usual conditions, some parts of the body are free from any kind of microbes, commensals or otherwise: these include the interior of the bladder (where the urine should be sterile), and the insides of the joints, where, similarly, the lubricating fluid should be totally free of micro-organisms.

Throughout the wider world, too, there are other micro-organisms living in balance with their surroundings. Many are to be found in the soil or on plants, and they are usually known as 'saprophytes'.

A 'pathogen', a term we have also used already, is a microbe which causes disease. Some always cause disease whenever they come into contact with man, but a more usual state of affairs is that they might or they might not, and this includes many which are normally commensals or saprophytes. Among such potential pathogens are *E. coli* and some varieties of staphylococcus and streptococcus, and saprophytes such as *Legionella*

pneumophila.

Whether microbes cause disease depends on the organism itself and on the human being concerned.

The ability of a micro-organism to establish the process of infection and produce disease is known as its pathogenicity. Pathogenicity varies considerably between one species of microbe and another, and this is obvious if we compare, for example, two virus diseases: chickenpox, caused by one of the herpes viruses, is quite mild, whereas rabies, caused by a rhabdovirus, is anything but. Further, there are differences in pathogenicity between strains (genetically distinct populations) of the same species.

Differences in pathogenicity are a function of the organism's invasiveness, which represents its ability to spread within the host and invade the body tissues, and its virulence, which is its ability to produce injury to those tissues.

The size of the infecting dose – the number of invading organisms – is also important, in that a large number of invading pathogenic organisms may overwhelm the body's defences, whereas a small number may be overcome or tolerated. In other words, a small dose of a highly pathogenic organism is relatively likely to produce disease, whereas a bigger dose of a less pathogenic organism would be relatively unlikely to do so. An experimental measure of pathogenicity is the 'LD50', which is the dose needed to kill 50% of an animal population inoculated with the particular microbe. The smaller the dose required, the more pathogenic the organism.

The pathogenicity of an organism depends either on the way it is structured, or on its ability to aid its advance by the production of toxins and similarly damaging substances. For example, whether or not a given strain has particular structural features (such as a capsule), or puts out a particular toxin, will help to determine its pathogenicity within a group. In recent years, an additional characteristic has been shown to be of importance: this is the adhesiveness of bacteria, their ability to stick to surfaces through which they then invade under-lying tissues.

The pathogenicity of bacterial strains may in part depend on genes which can be transmitted from one to another. It is known in the case of *E. coli*, for example, that both its capacity to produce toxins and its adhesiveness are determined by genes which can be carried between strains. This could help to explain some changes in the pattern of infection, such as the declining incidence of scarlet fever despite continuing throat infection by streptococci, and the less serious nature of staphy-lococcal infection of the skin in maternity units over recent decades.

Toxins

'Exotoxins' are highly poisonous polypeptides excreted by (mostly Gram-positive) bacteria which are still alive. They include the classical toxins of the clostridia, those of tetanus, botulism and gas gangrene, with doses of only a few micrograms (millionths of a gram) being lethal to animals. Toxins produced by various bacteria usually affect specific sites, such as the central nervous system or the heart.

Illness can follow ingestion of the toxin itself after it has been excreted by the bacteria, which is what happens in food poisoning by *Staphylo-coccus aureus* and *Clostridium botulinum*. The latter causes botulism; shortly after the person eats the contaminated food, the toxin is disseminated through the bloodstream and concentrates in the nerves of the head, where it thus causes the typical symptoms of visual disturbance and difficulties with swallowing and breathing. Toxins can also be produced inside the bowel by bacteria after they have been swallowed, and these may then give rise to purely local effects.

In other cases, toxins are absorbed through mucous membranes (as in the case of the diphtheria toxin from *Corynebacterium diphtheriae*, which is absorbed in the throat) or through wounds, espe-cially deep penetrating ones, the responsible organism in this case usually being *Clostridium tetani* and the resulting illness tetanus.

Bacillus anthracis, the causative organism of anthrax, uses an exotoxin to stimulate a massive flow of fluid and blood into the invasion site and thus facilitate spread of this highly pathogenic organism. Other Gram-positive bacteria produce exotoxins in association with related substances to promote invasion of the tissues; for example, the streptococci produce not only the erythrogenic toxin which causes scarlet fever, but also enzymes, streptolysins and leucocidins, which destroy defen-ding blood cells.

The other groups of toxins, 'endotoxins', are produced mainly by Gram-negative bacteria, and are the main factors determining their pathogeni-city. The precise structure of these toxins is not known, but it appears to be based on lipopoly-saccharides; what is known as Lipid A will, in doses of some hundreds of micrograms, be lethal to animals. They are usually released when the invading bacteria disintegrate and die, with effects including blood and fluid loss through the walls of blood vessels made newly permeable, shock, and coagulation of blood within the vessels. They also cause the release of hormones which give rise to fever.

Endotoxins are produced not only by bacteria which are almost always pathogenic to man, such as *Salmonella* (food poisoning) and *Shigella* (dysentery), but also by what are normally commensals, such as *E. coli*. However, when these commensals become the agents of opportunistic infection, it will be the endotoxins which cause most of the damage.

Capsules

When a bacterium encounters the first of the host's defences, it will be its possession or otherwise of a capsule which will be the most important factor in determining the outcome of the next stage in the battle, because a capsule will enable the bacterium

Mouth: saliva

Eyes: tears

Liver: bile
Stomach: acid

Airways: mucus & cilia

Skin: physical barrier

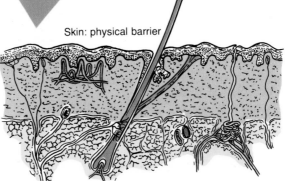

to evade many of these defences and thus become more 'invasive'.

Many virulent bacteria have capsules to protect them. They include *Haemophilus influenzae*, *Strep. pneumoniae*, *B. anthracis*, *E. coli* and *Salmonella typhi*, all of which use their capsules to resist attack by white blood cells whose function is to engulf and destroy them, the process known as 'phagocytosis'. Some capsulated bacteria even multiply within the white blood cells and are spread throughout the body in this manner.

Viruses as pathogens

The pathogenic effects of viruses depend less on the way they are made than on the response of the cells they invade and of the human body as a whole. Most gain entrance through the membranes of the respiratory tract or the intestines, but others penetrate the skin and mucous membranes or are injected by the bites of arthropods or animals. The next step is that they become adsorbed on to the surfaces of the cells, aided by specific features of the cell surface.

Some viruses remain at the site of the invasion and cause inflammation and local death of the surrounding tissues; others are distributed by the bloodstream and lymphatic systems to susceptible organs and tissues all over the body. Viruses may be specific to particular places (neurotropic for nerves, hepatotropic for the liver, and so on), or may infect almost any organ (pantropic).

THE HOST RESPONSE

Local and surface defences

The first line of the body's defences against infection is the mechanical barrier formed by the skin and mucous membranes, which provides good protection against the entry of pathogens and potentially pathogenic commensals into susceptible tissues. Fatty acids on the skin surface provide a further defence against those pathogens which require a neutral or alkaline medium, and the flushing action of tears and saliva helps to protect the membranes of the eyes and mouth.

Lysozyme is an enzyme present in tears, saliva

Figure 41 The skin, the mucous membranes and many of the body secretions form a barrier to infection.

and other body fluids. Its ability to kill (or 'lyse') bacteria was demonstrated by Alexander Fleming in 1922, seven years before he published his first paper on penicillin. Suffering from a cold, he showed that the drips from his own nose would destroy bacteria growing on an agar culture plate. After he found that tears had the same effect, experimentation proceeded only as fast as his associates could produce a sufficient supply by squeezing lemons into their eyes!

Among other natural body fluids known to have the ability to kill some bacteria are the bile and acids from the stomach's digestive juices. In the urinary tract, potential pathogens are washed away by the flow of urine. In the airways of the lung, bacteria are trapped in the mucous and then swept up and out by the wavelike action of the cilia, countless little hairs growing from specialised cells.

A few micro-organisms evade these blocks to their advance, among them being those that, like the malaria parasite, are injected through the skin by the stings of arthropods. Others go straight in through cuts and abrasions, the most important being those that cause tetanus and anthrax. And there are a few that can find their own way in through intact mucous membranes, notably *Treponema pallidum*, the causative agent of syphilis.

We shall describe antibodies in some detail shortly, but should mention here that a special

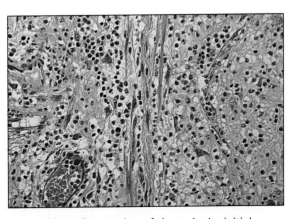

Figure 42 Inflammation of tissue is the initial response of the body to invasion by micro-organisms. White blood cells (polymorphonuclear leukocytes) migrate to the site of infection and impede circulation of the organisms; (magnification × 700).

variety of antibody, immunoglobulin A, is present in the secretions of the mucosa, and it probably helps to prevent invasion by stopping the micro-organisms becoming attached to potential host cells. Antibodies against the influenza virus can be found in the nasal secretions of people immune to that variety of flu, for example.

Micro-organisms which cause a particular type of disease usually find their way into the body through an appropriate portal; the airways, for example, in the case of organisms causing respiratory infection, or the mouth for bacteria which will cause diarrhoea by their action in the lower bowel. The body's defences are accustomed to such attacks, and come into action in an orderly manner. But when microbes attack in unexpected places, the consequences can be severe. A tragedy occurred in Australia in 1928 when a bottle of diphtheria vaccine became infected with *Staphylococcus*, and several children died when the bacteria were injected virtually straight into the bloodstream.

There are some areas of the body where bacteria never normally appear; they include the tissues of the brain and spinal cord, where even the supply of nutrients from the blood is indirect. If bacteria invade these parts of the central nervous system, very severe illness usually results, even though the organisms which most frequently do so are those that are the commonest commensals of the nose and throat and cause no trouble at all in their accustomed places.

The inflammatory reaction

Once bacteria have penetrated the skin or mucous membranes, a whole new array of defensive mechanisms come into action. The aim of these is to limit the spread of the organisms from the site of infection, to destroy as many as possible, and to wall off the site of invasion by fibrous connective tissue.

The first thing that happens is the provoking of the inflammatory reaction. The walls of the capillary blood vessels become more porous, allowing white blood cells (polymorphonuclear and mononuclear leucocytes) to pass through into the infected area; histamine is released from the damaged cells, dilating the blood vessels and allowing more blood to the area; and the lymphatic vessels become coagulated, impeding carriage of the bacteria to other sites.

The white blood cells, together with large specialised cells called 'macrophages', then set about the process of 'phagocytosis', and in so doing become 'phagocytes'.

Phagocytosis was a term introduced late in the last century by the marine biologist Elie Metchnikoff while working at the Pasteur Institute with starfish larvae. He noticed that if he stuck rose thorns into them, the thorns would become surrounded by 'wandering cells', or phagocytes, and this was despite the fact that the starfish had neither blood vessels nor a nervous system. He went on to observe and report on the way that fungus spores would become engulfed by similar phagocytes within the body of a water flea. We now know that antibodies on the surface of the phagocytes make it easy for them to stick to the bacterial cells which, once engulfed, are destroyed by enzymes (including lysozyme) within the phagocytes.

The byproducts of all this destruction, when in the presence of the white blood cells known as lymphocytes, stimulate the immune response, a physiological reaction of the human body which is of fundamental importance to a very wide variety of infection control measures. We will examine that shortly, but first consider what is perhaps the body's best-known, generalised response to invading organisms: fever.

Fever

Fever has been understood to be an accompaniment of infection since Hippocratic times, but until recently it was regarded as being an illness in itself, rather than the result of one. Learned physicians employed touch alone to determine the severity of the fever, and laid great reliance on variations in temperature – including the drama of the 'crisis' – to determine the course of the illness. Dr Thomas Southwood Smith, the anti-poverty activist and physician to the London Fever Hospital, wrote a book on fever in 1835 in which he suggested that there were several different species of the complaint, which he maintained was characterised by disruption of the nervous system and subsequent concentration of inflammation in one organ or another.

In 1888, however, Dr William Welch at Johns Hopkins University for the first time correctly related fever to infection by concluding that the raised temperature was the body's response to pathogenic micro-organisms and their products.

The normal temperature of the body is 37 degrees Celsius, or 98.4 degrees Fahrenheit, and in man it is maintained constant – save for normal small swings by night and day – by a thermo-regulatory centre in the hypothalamus of the brain. A rise in this temperature is stimulated by the effect on the hypothalamus of proteins called pyrogens, which are released by white blood cells following contact with bacteria and their toxins. Pyrogens obtain their effect by inducing synthesis of prosta-glandins in the hypothalamus, which is why prostaglandin inhibitors such as aspirin and cortisone reduce fever.

There are a variety of cells involved in the production of pyrogens, which explains why processes other than infection can cause fever. These include cancers, injury, and disturbances of the glandular and immune systems. In infections, the patterns of rise and fall in the graphed tempera-ture curve can give a clue to the disease. In some infections, such as typhoid, the temperature rises to a steady new level; in others, as when infection becomes localised in the form of an abscess, the temperature goes up and then swings wildly. In malaria, the temperature rises when each new batch of parasites is released into the blood, and as that happens at about 48 hour intervals, the fever occurs at those intervals too.

If an infection is untreated and left to resolve by itself, the fever either falls suddenly to normal – the 'crisis' so anxiously awaited in the days before antibiotics – or reduces slowly over a period of a few days.

The immune response

Once an invading pathogen has entered the body, it encounters three processes, all working together to combat and destroy it. One of these processes is phagocytosis, which we have already described. It is the main defensive mechanism available to the host who is not immune to that particular invader nor, for that matter, to any others. But to ensure survival, for the individual or for the species, this is not enough, and the development of immunity which is specific to particular invaders is imperative.

The other two processes are those that determine this specific immunity: one is cellular or cell-mediated immunity, and the other is humoral or antibody-dependent immunity.

The first principles of immunity were established in Metchnikoff's laboratories in the Pasteur Institute, and we have already noted that it was he who coined the term 'phagocytosis' to describe the activities of wandering and protective white cells. To the general concept, that in the body there are varieties of cells which attack and kill invading micro-organisms, he gave the term 'cellular immunity'.

By this time Louis Pasteur had already shown how suitably treated blood would kill the bacillus of anthrax and some other serious diseases. This and related findings were of course specifically related to infectious disease, but it was Metchnikoff's pupil Jules Bordet who, in a series of groundbreaking experiments, really established the science of immunology. This was to have implications extending far beyond the field of infection.

Bordet found that blood, with or without the cells that normally circulate in it, would defend the body against invading micro-organisms. Further, he observed that serum from blood previously exposed to infection – 'immune serum' – was more actively and successfully defensive in its ability to kill invading bacteria than serum from blood that had not been so exposed. During similar research at the Koch Institute at about the same time, it was shown that when cholera bacteria were injected into the peritoneal cavity of guinea pigs that had previously had the infection and recovered, the bacteria were destroyed by the peritoneal fluid, which has no cells at all in it. But the same fluid did not destroy bacteria other than those of cholera.

What Bordet and others had established was the concept of 'humoral immunity', and it was soon realised that humoral and cellular immunity were associated parts of the same defensive system. We now know that humoral processes are concerned with the interactions between antigens and anti-bodies, and the cellular processes involve the inter-actions between antigens and specialised forms of lymphocytes (one of the varieties of white blood cell), which take action directly as well as indirectly through the formation of other substances. Both lymphocytes and independent antibodies in the serum respond only to particular antigens, which they 'recognise'. This gives them their specificity, a feature of the body's defensive reaction which is not shared by phagocytosis.

The two categories of immunity are determined

by two different populations of lymphocytes, known as T cells and B cells. Both develop from the same parent cells in the bone marrow. However, the T cells (or thymus-dependent cells) are altered at some stage by passing through the thymus gland, and it is they that become responsible for the phenomenon of cellular immunity. On the other hand, B cells are independent of the thymus and are concerned with the synthesis of antibodies, the basis of humoral immunity.

Humoral immunity and antibodies

When the components of human serum were fully defined in the early 1940s, antibodies were found to be complex proteins in the gamma fraction of globulin. When these globulin molecules are acting as antibodies, they are also known as 'immunoglobulins', and receive the abbreviation Ig. There are five main structural types: IgG, IgM, IgA, IgD, and IgE.

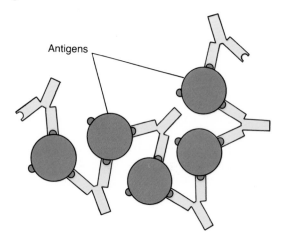

Antigens

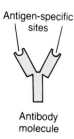

Antigen-specific sites

Antibody molecule

Figure 43 Antibodies link with invading antigens, facilitating phagocytosis of bacteria and neutralising toxins.

The body provides an extraordinarily wide variety of antibodies. What makes each one unique and quite specific in its action is the arrangement of the end parts of the chains of amino acids which make up the structure of the molecule. An antigen is a substance whose chemical structure is such that it can link and unite with the appropriate parts of the antibody molecule, such as these end chains.

The B cells which are carrying the antibodies are committed to responding to only a limited number of antigens. In the first encounter between antigen and antibody, known as the primary immune response, the B cells constrained to respond to this particular antigen proliferate by simple division, forming identical progeny with the now-familiar appellation 'clones'. Some of these become transformed into plasma cells, which are especially adapted for the synthesis and secretion of protein and become vigorous manufacturers of more antibody, which can then be set free into whatever is the surrounding body fluid. Other B cells become 'memory cells', which are programmed to respond quickly to any future encounter with the same antigen.

Among the antibodies, immunoglobulin G is the most abundant of all. It diffuses readily outside the blood vessels, where it is dominant in coating bacteria to facilitate phagocytosis and in neutralising bacterial toxins. It is the only immunoglobulin which crosses the placenta, and in so doing it provides vital protection against infection in the first few weeks of life. The transfer to the foetus occurs during the last three months of the pregnancy, so babies born before that time are deficient in the protection it provides and are therefore very susceptible to infection. The level of IgG in the blood falls after birth, but then recovers as the baby starts producing its own.

Immunoglobulin M is mostly confined to the blood. It emerges at an early stage after the appearance of antigen, and is effective in assisting phagocytosis by coating bacteria ('opsonising' them) and sticking them together ('agglutination'). It also works in association with another set of proteins in what is known as the 'complement' system, setting up yet another mechanism for the destruction of bacteria.

We have mentioned IgA in passing already: it is the antibody which is found in the secretions of those parts of the body which are exposed to the external environment, including the reproductive, respiratory and gastrointestinal tracts, where it assists the physical barrier of the mucous membrane to provide an early defence against bacteria and viruses.

Immunoglobulin E, like IgA, is secreted mainly in the linings of the respiratory and gastrointestinal systems, but it is concerned with allergic responses rather than with anti-infective activity. The function of IgD, which is at its maximum level during the childhood years, is at present unknown.

Complement, mentioned above in connection with IgM, is an important part of the entire defensive process. The complement system is comprised of a number of proteins which are usually activated by contact with antigen-antibody complexes, but which may also come into action as a response to bacterial toxins or the presence of viruses. A chain reaction occurs, which is highly destructive to the cell walls of bacteria and is also able to neutralise viruses.

Cell-mediated immunity

The cellular part of the immune system is mediated by T cells, and it is dependent on the presence of the thymus gland at birth. Children born without a thymus are very sickly, and die young. The lymphocytes which will become T cells migrate to the thymus and proliferate. Each cell is programmed for the antigens to which it will react, and they leave the thymus either to circulate in the

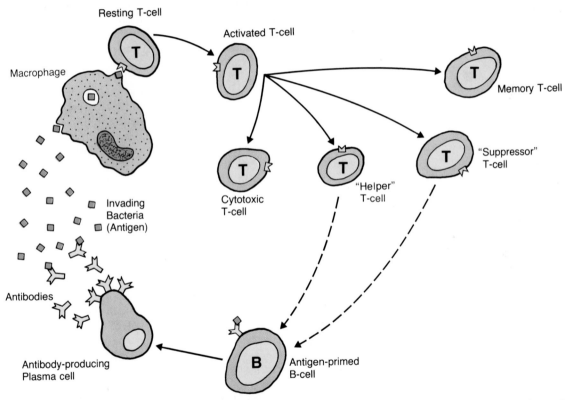

Figure 44 Invading bacteria are taken up by the macrophage and presented in a processed form to the resting T-cell. This causes the T-cell to become activated and reproduce into the following four specialist types:

(a) Cytotoxic T-cell which can destroy infected cells

(b) 'Helper' T-cells switch on the antigen-primed B-cells causing them to reproduce, forming plasma cells, which then produce antibodies specific to the invading bacteria.

(c) 'Suppressor' T-cells switch off the B-cells preventing overreaction and damage to surrounding tissues

(d) The longer-lived 'memory' T-cells with the same antigen-producing specificity are able to respond speedily to future challenges by the same antigen.

blood for about five years, or to settle in the lymph nodes or spleen.

Some antigens, including bacteria, immediately stimulate a cellular immune response when they appear on the scene. The T cells carrying antibodies to the particular antigen which is posing the challenge proliferate to form clones, and then differentiate into cells with different functions. All these descendants carry the same antibody receptors, but unlike B cells they do not liberate antibody into the surrounding fluids. Some destroy bacteria directly, and others become memory cells, increasing the number that will respond speedily to future challenges. Yet others become either 'helper' or 'suppressor' cells, whose function is to regulate the production of antibodies by B cells, preventing over-reaction and safeguarding tissues from self-inflicted injury by the powerful immune system.

PROTECTION IN PRACTICE

These, then, are the components of the body's defence forces, which provide protection against infectious disease. Bacteria are blocked at the outset by the natural barriers of the skin and mucous membranes, and are attacked by antibodies in the secretions on the surfaces. If they penetrate these barriers, they immediately encounter phagocytes, whose aim is to physically engulf and destroy them. Antibodies aid phagocytosis by coating bacteria and through the complement system, and the cell walls of the bacteria are broken down by yet more antibodies, thus exposing the interior to chemical disintegration.

From the infected patient's point of view, the overall progress of a bacterial disease is in most cases very different now, when compared to what he would have suffered before the availability of antibiotic drugs (see Chapter 8). In those days, the severity of the illness depended on the speed with which his body could bring enough phagocytes into action and produce sufficient antibodies to combat the invading and multiplying bacteria. In a fulminating infection, the bacteria might be able to outrun the defensive mechanisms, and this would lead to death. If, on the other hand, the antibodies prevailed, the 'crisis' would pass and the fever quickly fall.

In minor infections, this all still happens; bacteria entering through a cut are phagocytosed and countered by antibodies, and the site – marked for a while by the pus, which is all that remains of the cells involved in the encounter – is walled off from the bloodstream by fibrous tissue. When antibiotics are now used for more severe infections, they limit the number of bacteria which the body's natural mechanisms are called upon to combat.

Dangerous toxins are produced by some bacteria, as we have noted, and these dominate the infective process. The antibodies which inactivate such toxins are known as 'antitoxins' and, in the case of both diphtheria and tetanus, sera are made with the help of the horse in order both to treat the diseases and to prevent them (see again Chapter 8). In principle, of course, it is also possible to utilise for treatment an artificial 'serum' which would contain antibodies to specific bacterial infections, and indeed this has previously been done in the case of some pneumonias, but in practice antibiotic drugs are easier and safer to use.

When viruses attack, the body's defences are essentially the same as against bacteria, but there are some important differences. For one thing, an attack of some viral diseases – such as measles – confers immunity from the same disease for life, and this is a feature of those viral diseases which spread round the body in the blood. Others, generally those attacking mainly the surface membranes and having a short incubation period – such as the common cold, or influenza – confer some immunity, but not for long.

When viruses have been circulating in the blood they will, after the disease has resolved, have left behind antibodies and T cells which are already programmed for a fast response if reinfection should occur, with the effect being immediate defeat of any viruses which newly invade. The role of antibodies is to stop viruses entering susceptible host cells, and, in conjunction with complement, to assist phagocytosis and disposal of the invaders.

Thus, both the humoral and the cellular immune systems are also involved in the development of immunity to viral diseases, with their relative importance varying from disease to disease. Viruses of the common cold family attack the surface membranes; IgA antibodies will provide some protection against reinfection by particular viruses they recognise, but there are so many variants of the viruses causing respiratory illness that it is unlikely that a specific antibody will be ready and available for rapid action every time a virus lands.

Interferon is a natural protein which is another defender against infection by viruses. Interferon is produced by cells within two hours or so of becoming infected, and helps to prevent the spread of infection by diffusing into adjacent cells and preventing the viruses multiplying. It is active against many viruses and probably has an important role in limiting the spread of surface infections, and so its role in the treatment and prevention of viral disease is discussed in the section on chemotherapy.

Protozoa and metazoa also present a large number of antigens to their potential hosts, and can therefore stimulate a wide variety of immunological responses. The bodies of the parasites themselves may be antigenic, although this generally only becomes the case once the parasites die. Parasites may secrete antigens from the salivary glands or their equivalent during the feeding process, or release them from the anal or other pores. Both the B cell antibody system and the T cell system are involved in the immune response. The basic mechanism is the same as for the response to bacteria, but parasites are notable for their stimulation of non-specific immunoglobulins, and this might be due to frequent antigenic change, as occurs in trypanosomiasis and malaria. Another notable reaction provoked by helminths in particular is stimulation of a very high level of IgE, and although this fact is used for diagnostic purposes, the reason for and effects of this phenomenon are not clear at present.

Destruction of protozoa occurs in much the same way as for bacteria, but these mechanisms are of less use against metazoa. There are, however, some special lines of defence. Some larvae become coated with phagocytic cells, which so damage the surface of the worm that it dies. Cellular immune mechanisms may attack worms attached to the wall of the gut, so that they let go and are expelled.

In many worm infestations, an accommodation is reached between host and parasite. A moderate infestation sets up a moderate immune response, which helps to prevent the infestation becoming worse. And experiments have shown that it can sometimes be better to let the worms live; dead worms can be very antigenic and cause considerable damage.

Immunity

A person's immune response is not only concerned with the ability to resist infection, but also with other ways in which the body responds to foreign proteins, as in the rejection of grafted tissues or the wrong type of transfused blood. Immunity is determined genetically as well as through exposure to various antigens throughout life.

'Immune tolerance' is the capacity of the body not to react to some particular antigens. If such tolerance did not exist, the immune and complement systems would be constantly reacting to internal and non-threatening 'self' antigens, with highly damaging effects on the body it is intended to protect. Immune tolerance does sometimes break down (as a result, for example, of infection with some viruses, debilitating illness, or treatment with some drugs). This results in a state of 'auto-immunity', the end effects of which include the various forms of 'autoimmune disease'.

The foetus in the uterus lives in a sterile environment, and survival after birth requires the rapid development of antibodies specific to the antigens which the child is going to encounter. However, at birth the child will depend on the antibodies which have been supplied to it by the mother through the placenta, but as only IgG can take this path, the newborn is relatively poorly off for IgA and IgM. Further, as rising living standards have reduced the number of childhood infections, more and more mothers have developed fewer and fewer antibodies to pass on.

The IgG level falls after birth, and the child is particularly susceptible to infection at between three and six months of age. The speed of response to antigens is slower than at a later age, and the presence of some of the mother's antibodies to infections such as measles and diphtheria will further interfere with the newborn's capacity to deal with the relevant hazards. Further, the T cells are not at the time of birth capable of fully responding to challenge by antigens.

Soon, however, the antigens in the environment of the child will be programming the responses in a way that best ensures survival. It is as if a set of antibodies is waiting in the newborn body like an undeveloped photographic negative, ready for exposure to the appropriate set of antigens and development into a fully-fledged defensive formation. Just exactly what antibodies are already available at the time of birth for later stimulation is unknown, but by a very early age the child is able to respond adequately to most antigens he will encounter. In a study of antibody response among children in slum cities it was found that as early as the age of three years, most of them were immune to every common pathogen in their environment. On the other hand, children growing up in more sheltered and much cleaner environments are exposed to fewer antigens and thus build up fewer antibodies; it is a notorious fact of life in army recruitment camps that young adults coming from such a background are very susceptible to infection.

Immunity to disease falls into two categories: natural or inherited immunity; and acquired immunity.

Natural immunity may exist for an entire species, and the susceptibility of different species to infection varies widely. For example, mammals are immune to many of the organisms which cause disease in birds, and man is resistant to the distemper which is a risk to his pet dog. Sometimes,

few species are resistant to a given organism; salmonella, for instance, infects not only man but many other mammals, birds, reptiles and amphibians. In other instances, organisms are unique to one species; cholera and the gonococcus infect only man.

Fortunately, the human species possesses natural immunity to a huge variety of organisms which could produce disease, are all around in the environment, but do not.

A disease which can kill tends to eliminate from a given human population those who have a high degree of susceptibility to it. Thus, as generations pass, the inherited resistance of that population to the disease builds to a high level. Yet people living in remote areas who have never been exposed to the same illness – we have earlier mentioned measles in the South Pacific as an example – remain exceptionally susceptible to the same micro-organism, and the impact of exposure can be fatal.

Acquired immunity comes from exposure to

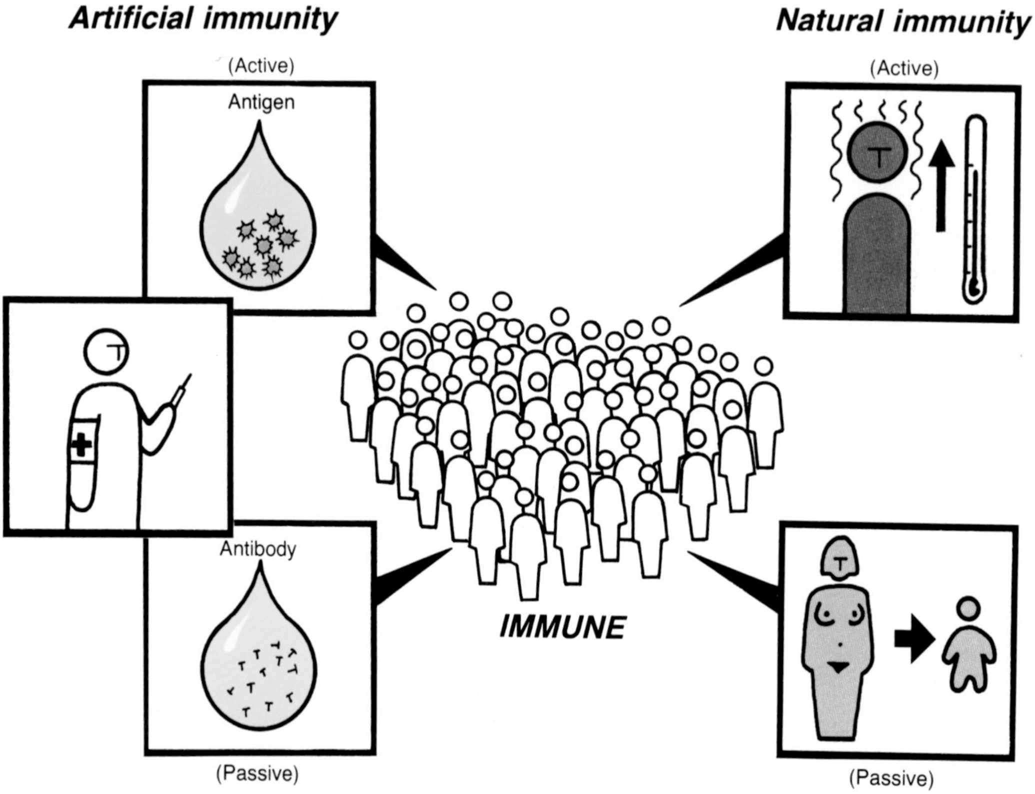

Figure 45 Immunity can be naturally or artifically acquired, in active or passive forms.

specific antigens. This can occur either as a result of having been infected by a pathogen, which is (confusingly) known as naturally-acquired immunity, or as a result of immunisation, which is artificially-acquired immunity.

Immunity can be naturally acquired *passively*, which is the process we have just described in relation to the way the mother passes immunity to the foetus through the placenta. This mainly depends on IgG. The baby's immunity therefore depends entirely on the antibodies that are in the mother's blood, and if the mother has no particular antibodies, the baby will lack them too.

Immunity which is naturally acquired *actively*, through response to infection by a particular organism, may result from a full-blown attack of the disease or from a sub-clinical and trouble-free infection by the same microbe. This latter is what happens in most cases as sturdy children build up their resistance to the wide variety of antigens they encounter every day, or people go to live for extended periods in areas of the world which are antigenically strange to them.

Artificially-acquired immunity can also be passive or active. Passive immunity, in this case, derives from the administration (usually by injection) of antibodies which have been produced by another host. The resulting immunity is instantly obtained, but only persists for a limited time, after which the individual becomes susceptible again. The antibodies may have been produced by a host of the same species (for humans, therefore, 'human immune globulin'), or by a host of a different species. 'Horse serum', for example, can be used to provide temporary protection from diphtheria and tetanus. However, in the latter case administration of the 'immune serum' is always open to the risk that the new host will react badly to it.

More effective in the long term is artificially-acquired active immunity, whereby antigens are deliberately administered so as to induce the production of antibodies by the host. In one example from days gone by, that of smallpox, live and unmodified organisms were employed in the inoculation, but since that time various methods have been developed to modify the organisms so that the antigens do not provoke a response which might be as bad as the disease. This whole process embraces the term immunisation, and is covered at greater length in Chapter 8.

Susceptibility

Infection does not equal disease. There are many factors which determine whether an infected person will become a diseased person, and the role of the immune system is clearly one of the most important determinants of all. But it is not the only one, and we shall discuss a few others at this point.

The *immune deficiency diseases* are a diverse group of disorders, characterised most importantly by an increased susceptibility to various infections. The consequence is that the affected individual suffers recurring and often serious bouts of acute and chronic infectious disease. The 'primary' immune deficiency disorders are genetically determined, with the individual being able to muster neither one nor both of the humoral and cellular immune responses. In some cases, there may be more specific deficiencies, such as in the ability of the appropriate cells to go about the business of phagocytosis. Almost any infection is dangerous for these people, and if the deficiency in T and B cell responses is absolute they rarely survive beyond babyhood. Less severe deficiencies mean a lifetime of fighting infection, and treatment includes as far as possible identifying the precise nature of the deficiency and rectifying it.

'Secondary' immune deficiency results from other disorders, including those stemming from kidney disease, cancer, malnutrition, the unwanted effects of some drugs, and therapy for cancerous disease. It can also result from infection by a newly recognised but already familiar organism, the human immunodeficiency virus, HIV, which causes the acquired immune deficiency syndrome, AIDS, now one of the world's new public health problems and described in the next chapter.

Genetic differences in susceptibility are almost certainly due to more than one gene, and we still do not really know much about the details, for example, of why one child in a group who contracts polio goes on to become paralysed, or why the HIV appears to affect different populations in different ways.

Ethnic differences in susceptibility appear to exist, but these are very hard to separate out from environmental influences, including cultural factors and nutritional status. Unequivocal studies relating malnutrition and infectious disease in man are hard to perform, because poverty, hunger and disease usually occur together in a self-perpetuating cycle, and because hunger is more common in places where severe diseases are endemic. Common sense, and the WHO, leave little doubt that malnutrition does contribute to the high rate of death by infectious disease in developing countries, that the populations in such places are more prone to infection, and that they suffer more when infected. In turn, infectious diseases have an effect on the nutritional state, and so the wheel rolls. Professor Thomas McKeown has argued that nutritional improvements were the main reason for improvements in the high mortality rates (mostly from infection, as we have seen) in the eighteenth and nineteenth centuries, but during the same period the general level of hygiene and sanitation also improved so strikingly that any uniquely nutritional effect is now very hard to disentangle.

Age, too, affects susceptibility in a complex and subtle manner. In poor areas with a low standard of hygiene, children who survive will do so with a wide variety of antibodies ready to fight off renewed attacks by pathogens, and subsequent infectious illnesses are likely to be short-lived and not severe. But in the developed, cleaner world, there will be more children who escape these illnesses in infancy, and when they first encounter the pathogens – at school, or as young adults joining large groups – the resulting sickness is liable to be relatively severe. This was apparent when polio was endemic – young adults who were infected were more likely to suffer badly, and become paralysed, than little children. The middle years of life are relatively free of the risk of infectious disease, as the antibodies are by this time well adapted to the antigens in the individual's environment, but finally, as the individual grows old, resistance falls along with the vigour of the other body functions, and infections – especially of the respiratory and intestinal tracts – become relatively likely again to cause disease.

6

The Spread of Infection

The control of infection demands some understanding of the balance between man and microbes in nature, the basic biology of the micro-organisms and the diseases they cause, the way that pathogens attack the body tissues, and the way that the body responds by activation of a variety of defence mechanisms. All these subjects we have touched upon so far. We have also examined the history of some measures that have been successful, and some that have not.

But modern control measures demand a further level of understanding, because they are so essentially based upon the way that diseases are spread and how the chain of transmission is broken. It is to these matters, therefore, that we turn in this chapter and the next.

GLOBAL PATTERNS OF DISEASE

Infectious diseases ebb and flow throughout communities, sometimes in gentle waves, sometimes like the onslaught of a tidal wave which causes terrible destruction before receding as quickly as it came, not to appear again for years. Patterns emerge and, inevitably, get given descriptive labels. To characterise patterns of disease we still use the names the Greeks used: epidemic, endemic, and pandemic. In addition, we even use the word sporadic, from the Greek for scattered, like the islands of the Sporades.

An *endemic* ('in people') disease is one which is always present to some extent in a particular community, geographic area or nation, with a steady but limited number of cases constantly occurring on a sporadic basis. Sometimes the term is used to apply to a disease (or, indeed, a plant) which is uniquely seen in a particular locality.

An *epidemic* ('upon people') disease occurs as an outbreak in a susceptible community, affecting an unexpectedly high number of people, but still within a specific area. What people characterise as an epidemic is highly variable, because it depends on the usual incidence of the disease in the region, and on individual perceptions of the severity of the disease and the threat it poses to the community. An outbreak of a handful of occurrences of a rare and serious disease might well be termed an epidemic, but many hundreds of cases of a familiar illness like influenza would be required before the same appellation was used in that instance.

A *pandemic* ('all people') disease is one which

occurs in what are perceived to be large numbers over a very wide area, a whole country, a continent, or even the globe. The speed of modern travel, which allows people to move thousands of miles while still within the incubation times of many infectious diseases, has added a new dimension to the possibility of pandemic occurrence of a disease. The explosion of influenza in 1918–19 was an example of a pandemic. Some people are calling AIDS a pandemic, not because the numbers even approach those of the 1918–19 influenza outbreak but because the level of perceived threat is generally very high and the whole world is under that threat. Clearly, there can be no hard and fast divisions between these three categories; one man's epidemic becomes another man's pandemic.

PRINCIPLES OF SPREAD

John Snow had no idea even of the very existence of the cholera vibrio when he showed how to halt the spread of cholera in London. In Central America, yellow fever was brought under control long before the virus which caused the disease was identified. It is not of critical importance to the control of infectious disease to know every single detail of the mechanisms involved in particular cases. Over the years, many reports and recommendations on disease control have had as their authors laymen who knew little or nothing about scientific method, let alone about the existence and life cycles of the microscopic agents of disease.

Nevertheless, the fact is that the more we do know about the way a disease is spread, the more likely it will be that our efforts to control it will be successful, and the more accurate that our knowledge is, the more precisely applied can our control measures be. An all-encompassing blunderbuss approach may well include some endeavours which do actually control the spread of a particular disease; but it may also encompass activities which have no useful effect on the spread of the disease in question, only serving to arouse the antagonism of the very people the control measure is supposed to benefit.

The principles of the spread of disease, around which the details can be built, are centred on the mirco-organisms. They embrace the various ways in which:

- they are liberated from infected people and animals, or from the environmental surroundings;

- they pass from the infected source to the new potential host;

- they enter the body tissues of the host and initiate the process of infection.

Successful micro-organisms will have an effective mechanism for transferring themselves and their offspring to other hosts. The microbes themselves may come from:

- among the commensals on the existing host's body;

- another person or animal;

- an inanimate object.

Factors affecting their spread include their ability to exist temporarily in what for them may be a hostile environment, and on their ability to survive and maybe multiply in places such as the surface of hands, bottles of milk or the bedclothes in a hospital. The number of microbes able to initiate an infection will be important, and this is of course related to the factor of virulence. They must be able to establish a portal of entry to the new host's body in order to set up the infectious process, and they must also be able to establish an efficient exit so that they and their descendants can go on and infect other people or animals.

Factors affecting the host which are relevant to the spread of infection, jointly representing the opportunity for transmission, include:

- the number of people in a given area and the proportion of that number who are susceptible to the disease;

- the proximity of the individuals to each other and to the source of the infection;

- the number of contacts these individuals have with each other.

The transmission of infection directly from one ill person to another is the most important form of spread for most diseases, and in the situations where there is no animal or arthropod intermediary – measles, for example – it is the only way the disease can be disseminated.

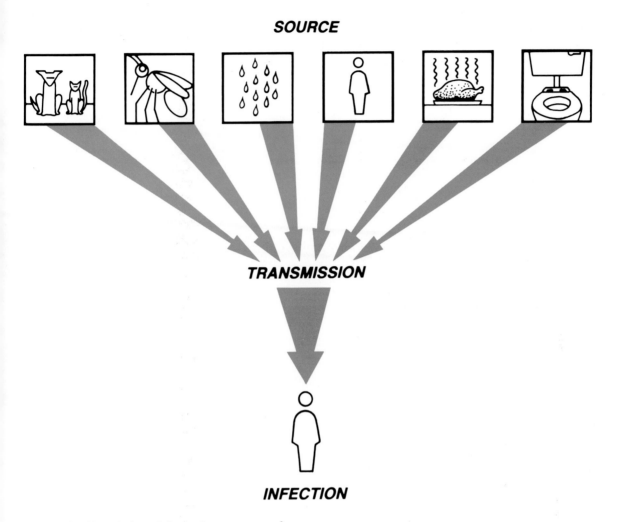

Figure 46 Knowledge of the various sources of infection enables us to control the means of transmission and thereby reduce the risk of infection by preventative measures.

The rate of spread of a disease depends in part on the interaction of the organism's infectivity with the opportunity for transmission. If one person infects five others, and those five infect five more, nearly 4000 people will become infected in five cycles of infection. The rate of spread also depends on the ratio of infectious people to susceptible people. If one infected person joins a group, all of whom are susceptible, then he will infect all of those with whom he comes in contact; say, one-tenth of all the group. They in turn will do the same. But on the assumption that infection will be followed by immunity, the time will come when most of the contacts of the infectious people are immune, and the rate of spread will drop sharply. If enough people in the group are immune, the infection will have a job spreading at all, an effect known as 'herd immunity'.

On the basis of the way infections are spread, they fall naturally into four groups.

The first of these groups includes those diseases which are disseminated by *faecal material*. Contaminated food and water are the most important intermediaries. These illnesses affect the digestive tract particularly; they include cholera, dysentery and typhoid, the diarrhoea of children, and some kinds of food poisoning.

The second group consists of those spread (highly efficiently) by sprays of *droplets* carrying the organisms, ejected into the air by coughing, sneezing, spitting or waving a handkerchief. The infecting organisms are commonly inhaled, and the diseases typically affect the respiratory tract. They include the common cold, influenza, measles and pulmonary tuberculosis, and these are all diseases where airborne spread is facilitated by crowding which forces people into close proximity. In fact, while aerosols containing microbes that float in the air undoubtedly transmit by the airborne route, those that are directly sprayed from a distance of a metre or less from person to person fall equally well into the next group.

This third group of diseases comprises those that are transmitted by *direct contact*, including the sexually transmitted diseases such as gonorrhoea and syphilis, and others such as herpes and tuberculosis. Contaminated intermediate inanimate objects, including clothes and bedding (known as fomites) can also distribute pathogenic organisms such as streptococci and staphylococci.

Finally, there are ·those which are *injected* through the skin into the flesh in some way. These include many diseases which are transmitted by intermediate vectors, usually arthropods or animals which bite or sting, and they include malaria, typhus, yellow fever, and rabies. They also include tetanus, which can be implanted in the flesh by a stab wound; and the HIV, which can be inoculated in a blood sample, and hepatitis B, which can be carried on an injection needle. Some protozoa also invade the human body by penetrating through the skin, the commonest examples being those that cause hookworm disease and schistosomiasis (see Chapter 4 for a fuller description).

All these represent what is known as 'horizontal' spread of disease from one person to another. 'Vertical' spread refers to the situation in which an infected mother passes the disease on to her unborn child, or to her baby during birth. Rubella is a well-known example, and in the developing world millions of cases of hepatitis B are also transmitted vertically. HIV can infect the child in utero and also possibly at birth, as can the organisms causing syphilis, cytomegalovirus disease and chlamydial disease. Among the most important

aims of the examination and screening of pregnant women are the identification and management of diseases which are spread vertically.

Reservoirs exist to provide secure places which are favourable for the survival of organisms and for their multiplication. Most pathogens are rather fragile creatures that are particular about the environment in which they are most likely to survive and prosper. Features they find most desirable are moisture, a warm temperature, the presence of nutrients and the absence of light. It is from such reservoirs that the organisms can emerge and attack man. Although soil (tetanus) and water (schistosomiasis) can act as reservoirs for some organisms, the reservoirs are customarily living organisms themselves, and the human body is the biggest and best reservoir and the most usual source of infection.

Many animals can also act as reservoirs for pathogenic organisms, and diseases of animals which can be transmitted to man are known as *zoonoses*. In Britain, these animals are most commonly favourite domestic pets or farm animals, and man becomes inadvertently involved with the relationship between organism and animal.

When a human – or, for that matter, an animal – is obviously ill, the danger to the community is less than if he is free of symptoms but acting as a symptomless *carrier*. Carriers are people who although not themselves showing any signs or symptoms of an infectious disease can transmit it to others. The presence of infection is unknown to all; the carrier feels perfectly well and may move widely throughout the community, thus ensuring equally wide distribution of whatever he is carrying.

Probably the best-known carrier of all time was a cook named Mary Mallon, who over a ten–year period cooked for eight different families in the United States at around the turn of the century. Denying she ever had the disease, 'Typhoid Mary' is known to have infected 54 people with typhoid, three of whom died.

People who are convalescing from infectious illness may still be able to pass on the disease from which they are recovering, although themselves feeling a lot better. Similarly hazardous to others are those who travel perhaps long distances within the incubation period of a disease from which they will finally suffer themselves, which gives them the opportunity meanwhile to infect a new population which may be very susceptible to it. This, indeed, was the very way in which some of the most terrifying epidemics of the past spread so rapidly, as people attempted in vain to flee.

Diseases which are associated with symptomless carriers, and those for which the responsible organism uses animals as reservoirs within a community, are likely to become endemic in that community and be very difficult to eliminate. One of the reasons that it was possible to eradicate smallpox is that it had no reservoir outside man; monkeypox, a closely related disease, which is fortunately only very rarely pathogenic in man, is endemic among monkeys and for all practical purposes could not be eliminated from the world in the way that smallpox was.

Vectors are the vehicles by which the diseases are carried from source to target. Most of the organisms which are most dangerous to man are carried by insects, the arthropods. Each vector has its own habitat, its own life cycle, its breeding season and unique sensitivity to various control measures, and all these have to be understood before control measures can be fully effective in limiting their numbers and thus controlling the diseases they are carrying.

Let us now examine some of the factors affecting the spread of disease, with a selection of examples, in a little more detail.

THE SPREAD OF DISEASE BY FOOD AND WATER

Diseases in this group mostly affect the digestive tract, and the responsible organisms are transmitted directly from human to human, or indirectly through contaminated food and water, or by insects. Not to put too fine a point on it, most of the microbes are carried in faeces. The control of this group of diseases in most countries, as we have described in outlining some historical aspects of the story of infection, has been one of the great triumphs of public health.

Faecal material may sometimes be carried virtually directly to the mouth in groups with exceptionally poor hygiene or little knowledge of hygienic concepts, such as children, and the infections can flash through an infants' school like a bushfire. Eating utensils, fingers and flies can all carry faeces, as can food and milk, but in poorer

countries the commonest intermediary is contaminated water. The pathogens involved may be bacteria, viruses or protozoa, and in all cases the disease process is set off by their being swallowed.

Typhoid

Typhoid has been over the course of history perhaps the most devastating of all of the intestinal infections. It has been known since Roman times, although it was not distinguished from typhus until the nineteenth century. The clinical features of typhoid fever were established during the mid-1800s, although for a long time it was one of the diseases believed to be spread in the air by smells and miasmas. We have already noted how it was that a Bristol general practitioner, William Budd, concluded after careful comparative study that the diarrhoeal discharges of his patients were responsible for the spread of the disease.

A feature of typhoid is the explosive nature of the outbreak once a food or water supply is infected. Only a small number of the infecting organisms are needed to produce disease and, as infectious disease generally in the Crimean, Boer and first world wars (in which more men died from infection than in battle), it had a calamitous effect on warring armies of the nineteenth century. In the Boer war, just as many soldiers of the British Army died from typhoid as from injuries inflicted by the Boers. In the American civil war about twice as many died from typhoid and malaria as from battle wounds, and in the Spanish-American war typhoid killed 1580 out of a total of just over a million Americans. This was over six times as many as died in battle.

By the turn of the century it was well recognised that every case of typhoid meant that someone had ingested someone else's 'alvine discharges', as they were known, and that in cities the prevalence of the disease was directly related to the inefficiency of the drainage systems and water supply. It is only during the present century that the incidence of the disease has dropped, and it has done so in an impressive manner, one of the most notable successes of the sanitary revolution.

But even in the best-ordered societies outbreaks still occur on rare occasions. In Croydon in 1937, 300 cases including 43 deaths resulted from infection of the water supply. In Aberdeen in 1964, 500 cases erupted from a tin of contaminated corned beef from Argentina. Even in Zermatt,

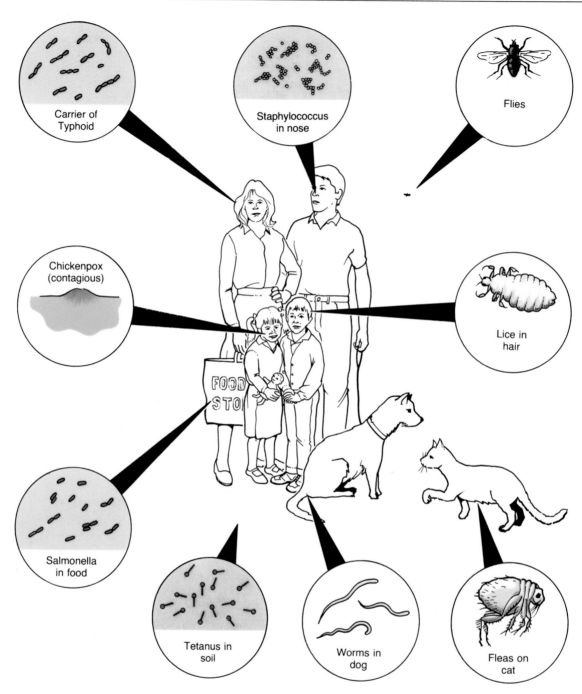

Figure 47   Reservoirs exist to provide secure places which are favourable for the survival of organisms and for their multiplication. The human body is the biggest and best reservoir and the most usual source of infection.

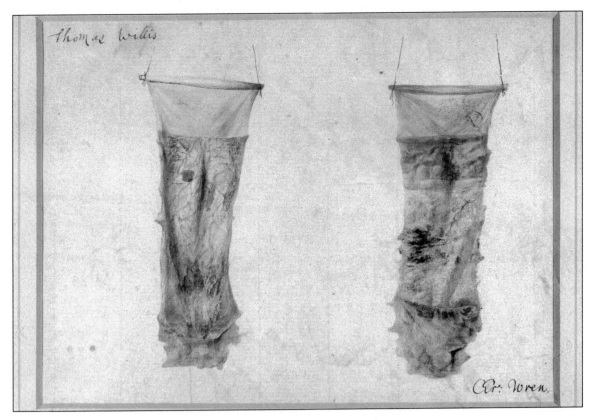

Figure 48   One of the drawings by Sir Christopher Wren of the ulcers on the wall of the intestine, a feature of typhoid fever.

Switzerland, no less, there was a sizable outbreak in 1963 caused by a contaminated water supply, and the disease was confirmed in 437 hapless holiday makers. As an interesting sidelight on the transmission of this disease (water-to-person rather than person-to-person), although over 70 holiday makers returned to Britain from Zermatt suffering from confirmed typhoid, only one secondary case is known to have ensued.

Typhoid and paratyphoid are grouped together under the term 'enteric fever', and are exclusively diseases of man. They are caused respectively by *Salmonella typhi* and *Salmonella paratyphi* (which is of three types). Salmonellae as a group are responsible for a very large number of gastrointestinal diseases, and more of them will be described in the section on food poisoning which follows. The name 'Salmonella', incidentally, has nothing to do with fish; the family of bacteria was named after Dr Daniel Salmon, who in 1886 first identified one of the group in pigs. Typhoid and

paratyphoid are very similar illnesses, although the latter is usually milder. The incubation period ranges from one to three weeks; then the infected person feels generally ill, as the bacteria become distributed all over the body. The internal walls of the intestine become ulcerated, a feature which was beautifully illustrated by Sir Christopher Wren as part of a series of drawings he did for a medical friend. The organism can become settled in the gall bladder and kidney and, as a result, be excreted in the faeces or urine by carriers who may continue to do so for years.

Typhoid is now very rare in western countries but is still a serious disease in parts of the developing world, although even in those poorer nations the death rate is much lower than it was because of the availability since the late 1940s of the antibiotic chloramphenicol. This drug, incidentally, is highly successful in treating the disease, but it does not prevent the development of the carrier state and it does not eliminate the bacteria from the gall bladder or intestines of established carriers.

Dysentery

Dysentery is a word which in many people's minds is synonymous with diarrhoea, especially that which follows the eating of polluted food. In countries like Britain the disease is not nearly as serious as it can be in the tropics, where profuse watery diarrhoea, with blood and mucous in the stools, can lead to serious dehydration particularly in children, and continued sickness for up to a month.

We are here concerned with bacillary dysentery, as opposed to the variety of dysentery caused by amoebae, which we discussed when describing pathogenic protozoa. Bacillary dysentery is caused by the *Shigella* species of bacteria, and is sometimes referred to by the less evocative name of shigellosis. It caused thousands of deaths in Japan towards the end of the last century, and it was there that Dr Shiga in 1898 isolated the causative bacterium, *Shigella dysenteriae*.

There are four main species of *Shigella*: *dysenteriae*, which causes the most serious illness but is confined these days to tropical countries; *sonnei*, which causes over 90% of bacillary dysentery in Britain; *flexneri*, the second most common in Britain; and *boydii*, again most regularly found in the tropics.

Sonnei dysentery is a common illness in schools and play centres for young children, as well as institutions for the old and the mentally handicapped. In all cases the spread is in faeces carried on the hands, and the organism is frequently found on toilet seats and associated hardware. Outbreaks can occur whenever people are disinclined to wash and dry the hands after defaecation. It can also be transmitted in food and water, especially where sanitary endeavours are poorly organised.

Cholera

Cholera is now, fortunately, of more historical than day-to-day importance. The bacteria, *Vibrio cholerae*, excrete a toxin which causes substantial loss of fluid, possibly exceeding half a litre every hour in the early stages. At this rate, death by dehydration can occur in less than ten hours, but the course of the disease is transformed by the administration of copious fluids.

Cholera is still a serious risk in the warmer countries, including the Mediterranean basin. Contaminated water and food, especially seafood but including anything that human excrement can find its way into, are the main sources. A vicious outbreak erupted in Naples in 1973, with raw mussels getting most of the blame, and the mussel beds in the polluted bay of Naples were destroyed.

Food poisoning

Food poisoning is a rather vague term, generally used to denote any acute gastrointestinal illness resulting from the recent consumption of food. It is essentially synonymous with 'acute gastroenteritis'. The period before symptoms occur ranges from only a few minutes in the case of some toxins, to maybe three or four days in the case of some bacteria. Then there is nausea and vomiting, abdominal pain, and diarrhoea. The symptoms are all too familiar, and there can be no person who has not suffered them at some time.

Food poisoning can arise from contamination of food by a wide variety of micro-organisms, including bacteria, viruses and protozoa, most of which have to be ingested in large numbers for illness to result. Despite all sorts of endeavours in hygiene and public health, the number of notifications and reports of food poisoning increased steadily in Britain during the period 1982–1986, and in 1986 outbreaks were – at 22,524 – the highest on record, with over 16,000 cases presumed to have been contracted in England.

Despite the fact that food poisoning is a notifiable disease in Britain, there is a huge difference between the actual incidence of acute gastroenteritis and the reported incidence. Accordingly, official statistics may simply indicate changes in the ways that the condition is being managed and reported. Nevertheless, it remains the case that foodborne enteric infections are among the commonest communicable diseases in the whole world, not excluding the most developed countries of Europe and North America. Estimated annual numbers of cases in the bigger countries run into the millions, and must represent a considerable drain on public and private resources.

There are many different kinds of food which can become contaminated. A few examples are as follows.

The flesh of raw meat from a previously healthy animal should be free of organisms, but it can become contaminated in two main ways. First, microbes which have been thriving within the gut of the animal can be transferred to the flesh during the process of slaughter and subsequent handling. Second, organisms can be transferred to the surface of the flesh from the environment, including dirty surfaces and hardware, and from the contaminated hands of people handling it.

Fish and shellfish may contain protozoa or toxins, and as shellfish filter huge quantities of water through their bodies they are particularly likely to harbour organisms if the water in which they are living is contaminated. During the winter of 1985–86 hundreds of people suffered from viral gastroenteritis after eating cockles from Leigh-on-Sea, leading to a complete review of the cockle-preparation process and a ban on fishing cockles from estuary waters known to be polluted. The flesh of some ocean-going fish such as mackerel and tuna can rapidly become toxic as a result of spoilage, causing the histamine-related symptoms of 'scombrotoxin' food poisoning – flushing, rapid pulse, sometimes diarrhoea and vomiting – very early after consumption.

Milk is a good medium for the growth of many bacteria; it is very likely to be contaminated if it is not pasteurised, but very unlikely to be if it is. Infection by *Salmonella* after drinking raw cows' milk appears to be increasing in England, but only a tiny handful of cases have followed the drinking of pasteurised milk, and these seem to have been associated with the mixing of raw and pasteurised milk in the processing plant. Milk powders have been found on occasion to be contaminated, perhaps because of contamination of the raw milk before heat treatment, contamination which is transferred to clothing or equipment and passed back to the milk powder during the later stages of manufacture. Bird droppings have been shown to contaminate milk powder plants, as have animal faeces adhering to the tyres of milk tankers.

Goats' milk, in many countries, is far less likely to have been pasteurised than the milk of cows, and may therefore be carrying a wide variety of organisms including those responsible for brucellosis and campylobacter enteritis.

Vegetables in the unwashed state are likely to have plenty of soil on them, and soil is a fertile source of many pathogenic bacteria. If vegetables are prepared on the same work surface as, say fresh meat, cross-contamination can easily occur.

Bacteria are the commonest infecting agents, with *Salmonella* and *Campylobacter* predominating. The members of the salmonella family which cause typhoid and paratyphoid have humans as the primary host, and as we have commented the organisms are spread either directly or indirectly (via food and water) from human to human. However, the natural hosts for the other salmonellae, which cause the vast majority of cases of bacterial food poisoning, are not humans but, rather, a wide range of mammals, reptiles and birds including poultry, cattle and pigs. Poultry meat is the single most important source of infection.

Most of the salmonella species are pathogenic to man, and more than 2000 types within the genus have been identified. Rather than go into complicated methods of classification (and the controversies surrounding them) it is more convenient simply to refer to the illness caused by them all, apart from typhoid and paratyphoid, as 'salmonellosis'.

Along with *Salmonella* species, another particularly commonly identified cause of food poisoning is infection by bacteria of *Campylobacter* species, with yet more including *Clostridium perfringens*, *Staph aureus*, *Bacillus cereus*, and *Vibrio parahaemolyticus*, the last two only having been recognised as causes comparatively recently. Also of comparatively recent concern (although very rare) is infection of milk and milk products by *Listeria monocytogenes*, which is a bacterium common in the environment. It has caused sporadic outbreaks associated with a high death rate, expecially in the United States and mainland Europe, and may not be destroyed by pasteurisation.

Salmonellae and *Cl. perfringens* are present in the intestinal tracts of many animals used for food, including pigs, cattle and poultry, and the surfaces of raw meat are therefore often contaminated by the time they reach the kitchen. Modern developments in the preparation of foodstuffs for sale have been blamed for increasing the risk to the community of salmonellosis, with for instance the intensive battery rearing of chickens and the recycling of feeds facilitating the spread of the salmonellae among the stock.

Surveys of mince and sausage meat have shown contamination rates of between 2% and 48%, and

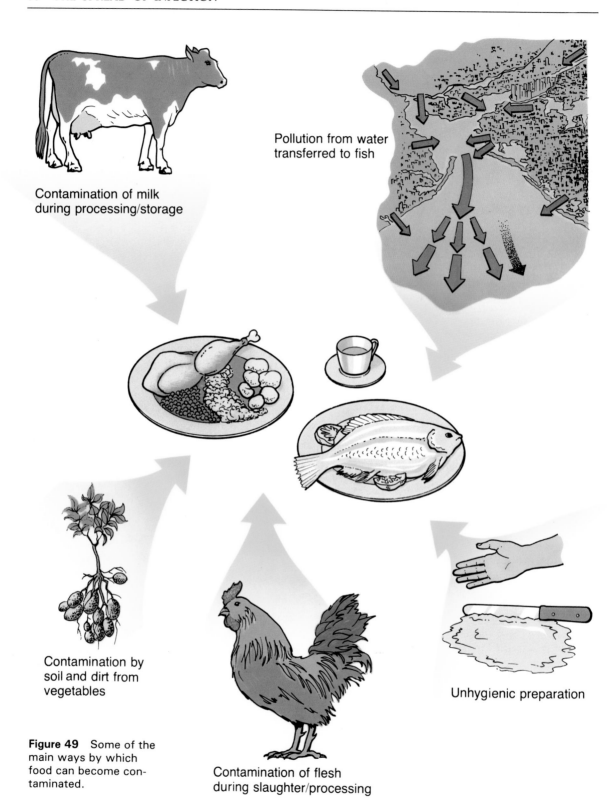

Contamination of milk
during processing/storage

Pollution from water
transferred to fish

Contamination by
soil and dirt from
vegetables

Contamination of flesh
during slaughter/processing

Unhygienic preparation

Figure 49   Some of the
main ways by which
food can become con-
taminated.

examination of frozen poultry has revealed contamination rates of up to 80%. Chickens and turkeys have been incriminated in 70% of salmonella outbreaks in England and Wales, although in some areas unpasteurised milk has been the medium of infection. Duck and hens' eggs are a source of salmonella gastroenteritis, because the oviducts of ducks can become infected with salmonellae, and the bacteria enter the eggs just before laying. Both chicken and duck eggs can also be infected after laying, with the bacteria passing through the shell as it cools while lying in infected, moist faeces. However, this is comparatively rare, at any rate in the case of chicken eggs produced under modern 'battery' conditions, because the faeces are dropped through grids clear of the new-laid eggs.

Inadequate cooking, cross contamination between raw food and cooked food, and poor storage of cooked food are what can result in ingestion of a sufficient number of the organisms to trigger salmonellosis. Outbreaks can occur under many different circumstances. Sporadic cases, occurring most commonly in the family circle, frequently involve lack of hygiene in the handling of raw meats, or inadequate cooking. At a hotel or restaurant, outbreaks involving groups of people can follow the eating of a contaminated meal, such as a turkey which has perhaps been left out, slowly cooling, for some time before consumption. Single cases occurring in a number of different households in a certain area may indicate that a supplier is at fault, perhaps in the way that he stores his frozen foods. Outbreaks in institutions such as hospitals and other health care centres are a special threat because of the likelihood of the contamination of food and the high chance that the contamination will then be spread from person to person on the hands.

The actual illnesses caused by the various bacterial causes of food poisoning have a similar nature, with variations in the severity of vomiting, diarrhoea, abdominal pain and general prostration. The majority of the bacteria bring about their effects by the release of toxin, which is released when the organism reaches the small intestine. In some cases the toxin is resistant to the heat of cooking. For example, heat-resistant strains of *Clostridium perfringens* form spores which survive cooking, and will subsequently germinate in meat or poultry which is allowed to cool to room temperature. Some strains of *Staph. aureus* also produce a heat-resistant toxin, with the contaminated food typically being cream or custard-filled bakery goods, but also including cooked cold meats and poultry, and seafood. The staph are likely to have originated in a food handler's nose or infected skin sores, and to have multiplied in improperly stored food.

Another member of the clostridium species, *Clostridium botulinum* (from the Latin *botulus*, a sausage), produces perhaps what is the most potent toxin and the rarest disease, 'botulism'. The symptoms are bizarre, because the toxin blocks the transmission of messages from the nerves to the muscles, and death occurs as a result of paralysis of the muscles of respiration. Antitoxin is now available, and treatment is usually successful if prompt. The organisms grow strictly in the absence of oxygen, and most commonly produce the toxin when growing anaerobically in meat-based food which is tinned. Heating the bacterial cells kills them, but they form spores which are extremely resistant to both heat and chemicals: boiling at 100 degrees Celsius for several hours (or cooking under pressure at a higher temperature for rather less time) is necessary to destroy them. The toxin itself is quite easily denatured by normal cooking, which may be one of the reasons why the disease is rare. Tinned food which needs no cooking, such as tinned salmon, has been the kind responsible for the most recent outbreaks of botulism.

During the depression in the United States many people turned to the home 'canning' (in tins or bottles) of meat. This led to a substantial increase in the number of reported cases of botulism, and much distrust of the home-canning process, which is dangerous if performed incorrectly. (The bottling of fruit and vegetables is a much safer process because their high acid content inhibits the growth of bacteria, including the clostridia.)

The role of *Campylobacter* bacteria (which have similarities to the cholera vibrio) as a cause of profuse and painful diarrhoea has only comparatively recently been recognised, and especially in the case of children there are suspicions that it may be the most frequent bacterial cause of diarrhoea of all. The sources of infection are the same as for salmonellae. *C. pylori* is a rather newly-discovered pathogen which seems to bring about changes in the lining of the stomach and duodenum leading to ulceration, so that this could therefore be yet another condition – not previously recognised as 'infective' – which may be in part caused by a micro-organism.

Another quite recently recognised cause of poisoning has been *Bacillus cereus*, the spores of which contaminate boiled rice when it is left out to cool, multiply and produce toxin. Quick reheating or frying the rice does not kill the toxin, and boiled rice should be refrigerated if leftovers are going to be eaten later.

The normal bowel is packed with bacteria including *Escherichia coli*, and every so often one of the strains which is pathogenic for humans causes an outbreak in a group; individual, sporadic cases are rare. Infection in this case is more of a problem for infants and young children, a fact which was identified following investigation of an epidemic in London in 1945 in which 21 deaths occurred among 51 children. Most of the severe outbreaks occur in hospitals or nursing homes, and breast feeding is the best preventive measure. An infant who is carrying and excreting the organism can very readily spread it to others, and in institutions, once identified, will normally have to be isolated.

Enteroviruses

Viruses, like bacteria, can be agents of infection carried in faeces by food, fingers and flies, and in temperate climes they are at least as important a cause of diarrhoea in infants as are bacteria. The term 'enteric virus', or *enterovirus*, is applied to any virus which is disseminated by faeces, and, like bacteria, they can be spread from one person to another either by direct person-to-person contact, or by water and food which has been contaminated by excrement.

Viruses excreted by humans find their way into water used for drinking. The public health significance of this has been hard to assess over the years, although bacterial contamination of water by faecal material has been a recognised possibility for a very long time. More than 100 different types of virus are known to be excreted in human faeces, and studies have shown that they easily survive many present sewage treatment methods, including chlorination, and persist for several months in natural waters. It is a fair assumption that where sanitation is less advanced, contamination is present and viruses are abundant. The presence of bacteria is usually taken as an indication of contamination of water, but viruses may be present in water which manifests little or no sign of bacterial pollution. Enteroviruses have been found in the rivers which act as the sources of drinking water in many cities of Europe, and wherever communities discharge their sewage into coastal waters there is the chance of contamination of seafood; viruses are inactivated much more slowly in the sea than are bacteria. Swimmers in polluted seawater or badly maintained swimming pools are at risk of ingesting contaminated water.

The best-known of the enteroviruses are the three types of polio virus, which can cause serious disease of the nervous system. The conquest of poliomyelitis is another of the more successful efforts of medical science combined with public health, aided on an international scale by the WHO. 'Infantile paralysis' was first described in 1795, and first recognised as an epidemic disease affecting the nervous system late in the last century. By sheer luck, the viral nature of the disease was identified by Karl Landsteiner in Vienna; luck, because the scientist used a monkey into which he injected nerve tissue from a fatal human case, and it was later found that the monkey is the only laboratory animal which can transmit the disease. A vaccine was developed by 1950 (see Chapter 8), and the incidence of the disease declined steeply between 1960 and 1970 in most western countries. However, almost inevitably, polio is still common in many developing countries.

During an illness which is rather like influenza, the virus travels to the brain and spinal cord; if the cells of the nervous system become damaged, paralysis can result, with a very wide range of severity. In the worst cases, rarely seen now, the paralysis affected the muscles of breathing, and the patient ended up in an 'iron lung' respirator.

In countries where the polio virus is still endemic, children have plenty of chances to encounter it and stimulate the formation of antibodies, so that the disease is not usually very severe and paralysis is exceedingly uncommon. However, if a person in or from the developed world now picks up the virus the disease, and the resulting paralysis, can be very serious.

Most of the other enteroviruses to have been so far discovered have come to light as a result of research into the polio virus. They include 'Coxsackie' viruses and 'echo' viruses, the latter getting the name 'enteric cytopathic human orphan' viruses because they were found in healthy chidren and were thus 'orphans' in search of a disease. The assumption was, at the time they were discovered, that the very presence of a virus in the human body meant that there must be an illness to go with it.

Most of the enteroviral infections affect children in the first few years of their life, and can easily be spread in households with poor standards of hygiene. They are highly prevalent viruses, about half of all children in preschool day nurseries having been found to be excreting them. Most of the resulting illnesses, when they do occur, are mild ones. In addition to gastrointestinal disorders, they sometimes cause respiratory disease and in such cases are spread through the air by droplets.

Yet another of the causative agents to have come to light in the last ten years, being apparently responsible for between one and two thirds of all infant diarrhoeas, is a group called the rotaviruses. This group causes diarrhoea of mild to moderate severity for a few days, sometimes with vomiting, and as with all cases of infant diarrhoea fluid loss can rapidly cause dehydration, which then needs urgent correction.

Although viral hepatitis, like brucellosis, is not a disease of the intestinal tract, it falls naturally into this section because one of the six or so hepatitis viruses is spread by faecally contaminated food and water. The different viruses cause slightly different forms of the disease, all with different names, the two best-known previously having been called 'infectious hepatitis' and 'serum hepatitis', but now referred to as hepatitis A and hepatitis B. It is the first of these two that we are interested in here; the other will be covered in detail in the section in which we describe the diseases spread by close contact.

The virus of hepatitis A is disseminated in the faeces and ingested by mouth in contaminated water and food, including meat, salad and shellfish. It is common throughout the world, especially in the warmer countries, and, as ever, is a serious public health problem where sanitary standards are low. It is apparently decreasing in incidence in northern Europe, North America and Australasia, all areas with well above-average standards of food hygiene.

The symptoms and signs of this unpleasant illness result from inflammation of the liver, with aches and pains and general malaise leading to nausea, abdominal pain, and the characteristic yellowing of the white parts of the eyeballs ('yellow jaundice'). People living in areas where hepatitis A is endemic become immune to it, and it is people who are travelling to such areas from places where the prevalence is low who are under especial threat. An immunoglobulin is available to provide protection, and is described in Chapter 8.

Apparently healthy food handlers, often during the incubation period (which can be from 15 to 50 days, and is typically about four weeks), can carry and spread the disease, which is sometimes therefore very hard to control. Shellfish can become contaminated in water where sewage is discharged, and vegetables grown with the aid of human faeces as fertilizer are potent sources of the virus.

DROPS IN THE AIR

Far and away the commonest and most important means of spread of infectious disease in the developed world is by way of droplets in the air, a route which gives rise chiefly to respiratory disease but also to a few other illnesses, including most of the communicable diseases of childhood such as measles and chickenpox.

Drops of saliva are ejected forcibly into the air whenever anyone talks, shouts, coughs or sneezes. Whatever the pathogenic organisms, and whether they are primarily settled in the nose, the throat, the airways or the lung tissue, some of them will be in the saliva and some of them will join this expulsive exodus. The bigger drops fall fairly rapidly to the ground, but the smaller ones float in the air in aerosol form, centred on dust-like specks too minute to see. The fluid part soon evaporates, but this still leaves a fleck of solid matter, complete with pathogens, to drift around invisibly. This fleck will take a very long time to settle, and will not leave the space unless propelled out of it in currents of circulating air which provide adequate ventilation. The nearest we can come to understanding such persistence is to watch dust particles highlighted by a shaft of sunlight, dancing in the air currents. If there is an infected person in any enclosed space breathing such particles out, then sooner or later anyone else in that space will breathe some of them in.

Fortunately, as will be clear to every reader by now, simply to breathe in a dose of pathogenic material does not mean that we will necessarily fall victim to the disease. All the body's natural defence mechanisms – including cilia, lysozyme, and IgA on the mucous membranes – will swing into action, and someone with influenza will probably only infect one or two other susceptible people before he recovers. If it were not so, we would all be ill all the time.

But even though we are not, the fact remains that about half all episodes of human illness are caused by viruses which infect the respiratory tract. Sickness from respiratory infections is the cause of about one-third of all the time off work in Britain, and the children of these workers suffer an average of about six infections of the respiratory system each year. Most of these episodes are mild, coming into the category of the 'common cold', but this still adds up to a great deal of disability throughout the community. Epidemics of influenza are the only outbreaks of infectious disease that nowadays, in developed countries, cause significant upsets in community life and short-term changes in the mortality statistics. Respiratory infections are essentially unconquered in the developed countries, unlike the major epidemic diseases of the gastrointestinal tract, and despite the effectiveness of the antibiotic drugs we now have against bacteria. In many undeveloped countries diphtheria is still a common cause of death. Vaccines exist for many of the childhood infections, but of all the common respiratory infections of later life only influenza has a vaccine available at present.

Practically all acute respiratory infections are caused by viruses, with bacteria only coming on to the scene as secondary invaders. Susceptibility to infection has been shown to be increased by exposure to tobacco smoke, including that inhaled directly and that inhaled 'passively' from a contaminated atmosphere.

The common cold

Numerically, the commonest viruses identified in people with respiratory illness are among the 100 or so types of 'rhinoviruses' and the several other viruses which are responsible for the common cold ('coryza'), regarded by the health professions (although not always by the sufferers) as a minor, self-limiting infection of the upper respiratory tract (which, as a matter of convenience, is held to be divided from the lower respiratory tract at about the level of the larynx). The illness takes hold after the viruses have become established in the lining of the nose or throat, from where they may spread upward or downward.

It is as well to stress, if stress is needed, that the common cold is caused and spread by viruses, although perhaps the fact that this was not proved until the 1930s is the reason for so much widespread misconception now. The London lecturer on medicine, Thomas Watson, may have introduced the word 'cold' into the literature and common parlance in this context in his 1853 lectures on the Principles and Practice of Physic, wherein, discussing 'catarrh', he commented that 'Not one man in ten thousand passes a winter without having a cold of some sort . . .', and went on to suggest that it was caused by cold and wet air on the skin.

In the United States colds were for the first time successfully passed from person to person by bacteria-free filtrates of nasal secretions in 1930, but no virus was identified. In Britain the Common Cold Research Unit was established just before the second world war, and over the next few decades made it clear that colds were caused by an amazing array of different viruses, which was gloomy news for those who had hoped for a single vaccine to prevent them. The Unit made a great many people very uncomfortably cold and wet during the course of their research, and showed that no such miserable environmental conditions were ever able to 'give them a cold'.

Research on the way colds are spread, therefore, and the proof of their disparate viral causation, shows at least four things:

- antibacterial drugs will neither prevent nor cure an uncomplicated cold;

- no vaccine is ever likely to be available to prevent colds;

- the environment does not trigger colds, viruses do;

- the situation most effective for transmitting colds is the close proximity of lots of people in poorly ventilated enclosed spaces, an all too common set of circumstances in the British winter.

Apart from the general misery and economic hardship posed by colds, the main threat to health is through the onset of complications, caused mostly by bacteria invading tissues in and around the upper respiratory tract which have been laid open to attack by the inflammatory reaction set off by the virus. These complications include otitis media, infection of the middle part of the inner ear; tonsillitis and pharyngitis, often from the invasion of streptococci; and sinusitis, with headache and pain in the bones of the face.

Lower respiratory infections

In the lower respiratory tract, several different bacteria play their part in causing infectious disease. *Streptococcus pneumoniae* is the dominant cause of pneumonia in adults and, with pneumococci, poses a particular threat to the elderly, those with pre-existing chest disease and those who are smokers. In children, inflammation of the medium-sized air passages in the lungs, bronchiolitis, can be alarming and sometimes dangerous; it is often caused by a fairly newly-discovered virus, respiratory syncytial virus, and tends to occur in autumn epidemics.

Influenza

Influenza is one of the most interesting of all the diseases which are spread by droplets of saliva. Not only has it been responsible for some of the most lethal pandemics of all time, it is still the only one of the great epidemic diseases not to be under global control. Yet, perhaps because almost everyone has personal experience of it, its name does not have the fearful connotations of other infections such as, say, leprosy or rabies.

Until the last century or two, it was just yet another of the many afflictions of mankind, and not, in comparative terms, even a very severe one. Charles Creighton, the great historian of epidemics, suggests two possible origins for the name 'influenza', one originating from ancient humoral concepts of pathology, 'influxio', meaning catarrh; but it is the other which has more widespread acceptance now, influenza being the Italian word for 'influence', perhaps of the stars or perhaps of the cold. 'La grippe', the French term for the illness, was the name given to a common insect which was supposed to bring about an epidemic by contaminating the atmosphere.

There have been scattered references to the disease since the twelfth century, recognisable from descriptions of symptoms and, more reliably, from the characteristic pattern of the outbreaks. By the eighteenth century the disease was being faithfully described by English doctors, and historians are now able to piece together a historical record which shows the irregular but frequent appearance of pandemics sweeping Europe and in some cases the entire world.

Typically, the pandemics spread from the east: that of 1781–82, for example, appeared first in Asia and spread through Russia, reaching north and east Europe about six months later and going on to southern Europe. London was struck, although not very badly, in June 1782, and as in the horrendous pandemic of 1918–19 the illness concentrated its effects on young adults rather than children and the old. Similarly, the pandemic of 1847–48 was in Russia in March 1847 and reached England in the winter. This was a bad one, and affected the elderly in particular; during a six-week period, about 5000 people died directly or indirectly from its effects. Creighton comments that as in all influenza epidemics of that and earlier times, the rich were as affected as the poor; although sheltered as they were from the dreadful sanitation and filth which killed so many of the poor people from intestinal disease, they had no such protection against this most democratic of epidemics.

The pandemic of 1889–93 was the one during which for the first time the typical wavelike nature of the incidence of influenza was recorded. The first wave was not very severe, but the other three waves were each responsible for the deaths of more than 2000 people in London, again predominantly young children and the elderly. It was during this pandemic that a bacillus was found so frequently in the lungs of victims that for many decades, with some controversy, it was assumed to be the causal agent and was named *Haemophilus influenzae*.

The 1918–19 pandemic was one of the worst worldwide outbreaks of disease of all time. It afflicted more people, and had a higher death rate, than any other epidemic disease since the Black Death, six centuries before. It has been estimated that a total of about 22 million people died, including about 150,000 deaths in Britain and half a million in the United States. The death rate was much higher in some remote countries, with the highest mortality rate of all being recorded in Samoa, where one-quarter of the entire native population succumbed to influenza.

This pandemic, typically, came in waves. From

Europe (possibly from Spain – it is not known for sure where this pandemic originated) in the spring of 1918, a mild ·epidemic struck England in the summer, but surged back again later in the year, with the highest mortality in November and December, and a resurgence in the early spring. The spread was at lightning speed: new cases were reported simultaneously on opposite sides of the globe. A striking difference from most earlier pandemics was that on this occasion the death rate was exceptionally high among young adults, who usually fared rather better than their younger and older contemporaries.

The war must have had its effect, in Europe at least. Young men were packed together in massive concentrations in generally poor living conditions, and together with the upheaval in normal society, the circumstances were favourable for the spread of any infectious disease.

This pandemic, and the less devastating ones which followed· it, stimulated worldwide research on the cause of 'the influence'. In 1933 filtered material from the nasal secretions of sufferers in England was used in an attempt to reproduce the disease in all conceivable laboratory animals; the usual ones, such as rabbits, guinea pigs and mice simply did not get flu. It was known, however, that ferrets were susceptible to distemper, the viral disease of dogs which is very similar to influenza, and sure enough they did develop the disease. This at last made systematic research possible; soon afterwards it became possible to culture the virus in chick embryos, and the various types of influenza virus were isolated for the first time.

There are three main types of influenza virus: A, B, and C. Type A is essentially a disease of animals, as it infects many birds and animals as well as man. Types B and C appear only to infect man, but C is rarely found. Type A virus has the ability to change its antigenic nature, with major changes in the surface antigens – 'antigenic shift' – enabling the virus to overcome established herd immunity and cause regular new epidemics and pandemics.

One such major change occurred in the case of the 1957 pandemic of 'Asian flu'. During the winter of 1956–57 influenza appeared in China, but because China was not a collaborator in the worldwide system of Influenza Surveillance Centres which had been set up by the WHO, few people knew about it until epidemics occurred in Singapore and Japan, later to spread round the

world and recur in a series of waves as one of the most widespread pandemics ever. In southern China, as in other parts of Asia, people live in close association with pigs and ducks, both of which act as hosts to the influenza virus, and it has been suggested that periodically a process of natural genetic recombination occurs, involving the animal and human reservoirs. In addition, both types A and B show the capacity for 'antigenic drift', whereby minor variations become selected out as the most successful mutations in particular epidemics, giving rise to the observed steady changes in antigenic nature over the years.

The aim of the WHO Influenza Surveillance Centres is to recognise the existence of, and isolate, any new strain of virus which emerges in time for a vaccine to be prepared against it. Nevertheless, whenever there are large numbers of non-immune people in a given community, and a suitable strain of virus appears, an epidemic is likely. Indeed, so efficient is the virus at spreading that if an epidemic occurs anywhere in the world, it is a fair bet that within a year any other susceptible populations elsewhere in the world will have suffered an epidemic caused by the same strain of virus.

Tuberculosis

Epidemics of short-lived, fast-spreading and spectacular illnesses, with sufferers either dying or not and the issue settled one way or the other within a few days, have quite naturally received the lion's share of public regard over the centuries. Yet it was a disease whose every process is slow, and with resulting deaths occurring after a lingering sickness, that over the years killed more people than any of its more dramatically-paced contemporaries; truly, as Bunyan called it, 'Captain of all the men of death'. The disease, of course, is tuberculosis.

Not that the disease has been free of its own kind of drama. Keats, himself suffering from tuberculosis, wrote in 1819 that 'youth grows pale and spectre thin and dies', and the pale features of the sick promoted the name 'the white plague'.

The tubercle bacillus, *Mycobacterium tuberculosis*, is coughed up by the sufferer and expelled in saliva droplets, to be inhaled in the way typical for the group of diseases being discussed. The surface of the bacillus has a waxy coating which slows the rate at which it multiplies, protects it to some extent from phagocytosis, and sets up an

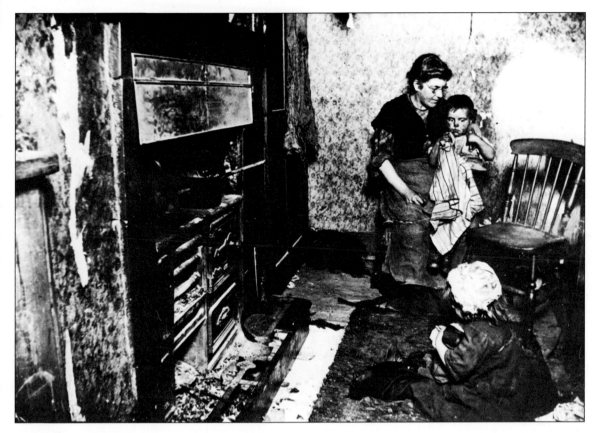

Figure 50 Damp and insanitary housing conditions contributed greatly to the incidence of diseases such as tuberculosis.

inflammatory process which is – like most features of this disease – slow in action. Simple and shortlived inhalation is on its own relatively unlikely to set up a new full-blown infective process; even when a small spot of tuberculous inflammation is set up in the lung, it only rarely develops into widespread disease. To an extent, then, by the standards of influenza and the common cold, it is not that infectious.

The incidence of tuberculosis reflects living conditions and standards – especially such features as overcrowding and poor ventilation – far more accurately than other droplet-spread infections do, because for the disease to spread, infectious people have to be in close proximity to susceptible potential hosts for extended periods.

Thus, well before drugs became available to treat the disease, its incidence was falling in countries where living standards were improving.

In Britain and most western nations most of the cases and most of the deaths are now among immigrants, the chronically ill and the elderly, especially those who have a drinking problem and are down and out. Surveys using skin tests have shown that many of these old folk must have been infected as children and have carried the infection ever since, with frank disease only breaking out under the influence of deprivation, malnutrition and alcohol.

Immigrants have consistently been among the worst-affected groups, but they have commonly brought tuberculosis with them from their home countries. The spread of the disease within immigrant communities has reflected the living conditions which they have so often had to face in their adopted lands. Irish immigrants to America suffered badly; but tuberculosis was also common in Irish cities, and it was not a unique susceptibility to the disease which caused the illness in their new land, it was being crowded together in an atmosphere heavy with the tubercle bacillus. Similarly, the coloured people of the United States now have a higher incidence of tuberculosis; but records show that the disease was uncommon among slaves, who lived generally in better conditions, and with a better diet, than they faced after emancipation and their mass migration to the cities.

Robert Koch demonstrated the cause and method of spread of the tubercle bacillus in 1882, but some 20 years earlier a French army surgeon, Jean Villemin, had transmitted tuberculosis from animal to animal by inoculation, and Dr William Budd (of typhoid fame) had suggested that tuberculosis was one of a number of diseases spread by matter cast off by sufferers and disseminated under crowded conditions; he cited as examples prisons, ships, convents and (of all things) harems.

Although most tuberculosis is spread by droplets and affects the lungs, it is a disease of the whole body and can also be spread by direct contact and by vectors such as milk. Cattle were known to be an important reservoir of the disease by the turn of the century, and surveillance of both animals and man was accelerated after the finding that most of Queen Victoria's dairy cows, renowned as the cleanest herd in the land, had the lesions of tuberculosis. Tuberculosis of cattle has been eradicated in Britain and similarly developed countries by various control measures, including the testing of milk and the slaughter of infected animals.

The slow, insidious spread of the disease was a reason for the success of the sanatorium programme, separating out from the rest of the community those who were the most infectious. The introduction of drug treatment, and the controversial use of vaccines, are subjects discussed later, when control measures are considered in more detail.

Tuberculosis is still a common disease in the developing countries, especially in South-East Asia and Africa. Although the decline in developed countries is at the rate of around 14% each year, in Britain nearly 6000 new cases were notified in 1986.

Communicable diseases of childhood

Most of the communicable diseases of childhood are spread by the respiratory route, and their control has been one of the primary medical achievements of the twentieth century. Diphtheria, for example, is a serious illness, and was at one time the most common of all childhood diseases. As a result of widespread immunisation it is now rare in Britain, but in many poor countries diphtheria is still a common cause of deaths. The mortality from measles, a highly infectious ailment, has fallen steeply since the turn of the century to its presently very low level; nevertheless, it still causes considerable sickness. Over 80,000 cases are reported each year in the UK, with many thousands more not being notified, and it is a continuing cause for concern in the tropics and remote corners of the world. Rubella, or German measles, is a mild complaint except for its potential effect on the newborn, which can be circumvented by immunisation. Chickenpox, yet another highly infectious disease of worldwide distribution spread by the droplet route (it has also been transmitted experimentally by the fluid in the vesicles) is currently regarded on the one hand as so infectious, and on the other as causing so little significant morbidity, that there is not really any point in trying to prevent it.

The principles of immunisation will be considered further in the next chapter; the most important point to be made here, in the context of infection control generally, is that immunisation is the only practical way of controlling most respiratory diseases spread by the droplet route, and if there is no way of immunising people, the disease in question is likely to remain endemic.

CONTACT AND CONTAGION

The third method by which infection is spread is through close bodily contact between humans, once more commonly referred to as 'contagion' and 'contagious disease'.

The sexually transmitted diseases make up the bulk of this group, and in addition there are some illnesses found mostly in tropical areas which are also spread by close personal contact. These include the eye disease trachoma, carried to the eyes by contaminated fingers, cloths and so on. In addition, it is convenient to include within this category that large group of infections which arise within, and are spread around, hospitals and other health care centres, because the mode of spread is predominantly (although not exclusively) through contact with infection-carrying hands and various pieces of medical paraphernalia, bedding and the like.

Medical science has had by the general standards of recent years a disappointing record in getting to grips with sexually transmitted disease (a term now used in preference to the traditional but less precise 'venereal disease'). The number of pathogens now known to be sexually transmitted exceeds 20, including one which appears to be inevitably fatal. The 'classic' sexually transmitted diseases, such as syphilis and gonorrhoea, are now under reasonable control in the developed countries, but are increasing in incidence in other parts of the world. Further, sexually transmitted diseases in a 'second generation' wave are tending now to replace the older ones in both importance and frequency; not only that, but those in the new group are harder to identify, treat and control. The late complications of the sexually transmitted diseases appear to be increasing the incidence of associated conditions such as chronic inflammation of the pelvis, pregnancies occurring outside the uterus, infertility and carcinoma of the cervix.

Sexually transmitted diseases pose a special threat to the developing world because of demographic changes. In the industrialised countries, the 'baby boom' is over; relatively speaking, it is the number of people in the older age groups that is increasing. But in the developing world the birth rate remains high, so that as a given population increases in size it does so particularly among children and young adults. And it is young adults who are most at risk from sexually transmitted disease.

Syphilis and gonorrhoea

Both syphilis and gonorrhoea have been acknowledged for centuries, but the histories of the two conditions tend to be merged because of much perplexity on just how many sexually transmitted diseases were responsible for the observed symptoms; further, there used to be much confusion with leprosy and smallpox. For example, Creighton quotes an Ordinance of Edward III addressed to the Mayor and Sheriffs of London, in which it is stated that lepers communicated their disease by 'carnal intercourse with women in stews and other secret places', so that it is not at all clear whether the disease under such censure was actually leprosy or syphilis.

Syphilis became only too apparent in Europe as the result of pandemic spread of a virulent form of the disease which started in the later years of the fifteenth century. It coincided with the return of Columbus and his men from the New World, which accordingly took the blame as the point of origin; but it is at least as likely that the venereal form of the disease evolved as a result of the mutation of related organisms known to have been responsible for endemic non-venereal diseases in Africa and Asia for thousands of years before.

Syphilis received its name from Girolamo Fracastoro, who in 1530 wrote a long poem, *Syphilus sive Morbus Gallicus*. This describes how the shepherd Syphilus aroused the ire of Apollo, who bestowed painful ulcers on his body:

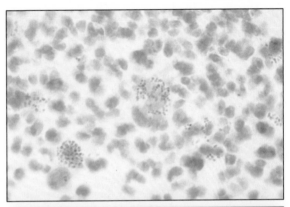

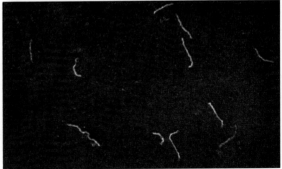

Figure 51 The routes of transmission of sexually transmitted diseases are now known and thus, in principal, the way to control them. But in practice, human co-operation and changes in behaviour are required which may be difficult to achieve.

(a) Gonococcus, the causative organism of gonorrhoea

(b) Spirochaete of syphilis

'And soon a vicious ulcer eats its way
Into the privates. And a vengeful sway
Takes cancerous possession to remain
Extended to the groin is its fell bane'.

But still syphilis and gonorrhoea were confused. In a heroic but thoroughly ill-advised experiment in 1769, the great surgeon John Hunter inoculated himself on the penis with matter from a gonorrheal discharge, 'proving' to his satisfaction that this would cause a (syphilitic) chancre, or ulcer. But because the matter had come from a patient with both gonorrhoea and syphilis the confusion was simply confounded. It was not until the late nineteenth century that the bacilli causing gonorrhoea and syphilis were separately identified, and the two diseases systematically described.

The number of people with syphilis newly attending special clinics in England now totals around 1000 each year and is currently falling, a trend which has become particularly pronounced in younger males only since 1985.

Gonorrhoea, which is far commoner, is caused by the gonococcus *Neisseria gonorrhoeae*. About 46,000 cases are now reported in England each year. It causes inflammation of the urethra and associated tissues, and the long-term complications can be serious, including stricture of the urethra in men and infertility in women.

The causative organism of syphilis is a corkscrew-shaped spirochaete, *Treponema pallidum*. Untreated, this causes ulceration (chancres) of the genitalia after about three weeks, and a general malaise and fever some two months later. Once over these symptoms the individual may feel quite well, but still has 'latent' syphilis. In some cases, years later again, a wide variety of complications may become apparent, including involvement of the nervous system and mental disturbance. Syphilis is at its most infectious in the early stages, and after a period arbitrarily taken as about two years the disease is no longer infectious.

There has been a steady decline in the reported incidence of gonorrhoea, with different trends at different ages. The decline in the disease among those of both sexes has been greatest at older ages, and the steepening in the decline which has become apparent in males aged over 35 since 1982 may represent a change in behaviour among homosexual men following publicity about the risk of AIDS infection. However, there has been no such recent decline in males and females aged from 16 to 19 years, and in fact the comparatively high rate among these groups increased slightly during 1985.

Both the cause and the routes of transmission of syphilis and gonorrhoea are known, we know how to test for them at an early stage, and both are diseases which are confined to man. Both are, therefore, in principle eradicable. But the fact that both still strongly prevail points to the special difficulty of bringing under community control diseases spread by close – intimate, that is – personal contact, with all the social implications that arise from this reality.

These two diseases are joined today, as we mentioned above, by the second generation of sexually transmitted diseases. They include infection by the bacterium *Chlamydia trachomatis*, the human herpes viruses, the human papilloma viruses, the virus of hepatitis B, and the virus of the acquired immune deficiency syndrome (AIDS). They can all cause chronic ill health and disability, even death. In addition to these, there are a few pathogens which nobody until recently even knew could be transmitted sexually, including for instance intestinal parasites passed from person to person by anal-oral contact.

Most reasonably accurate information on the incidence of sexually transmitted diseases arises from studies and routine statistics in the developed countries, and even these figures have a degree of unreliability which depends on the accuracy of reporting, something which is especially problematical in the case of maladies of this nature. In any event, what the reported figures show is that in these countries, gonorrhoea is still rising in incidence, although a rapid rise which was seen in the 1960–80 period appears to have slowed. Reported gonorrhoea has increased more among women than men. The incidence of reported syphilis is much lower than that of gonorrhoea; the disease has come and gone over recent years in gentle waves, and is commoner in men (mostly homosexual men) than women.

Infections by *Chlamydia* are now known to be the biggest single cause of urethritis not caused by the gonococcus, and in Britain non-gonococcal urethritis, having risen in reported incidence very steeply, is now more than twice as common as gonorrhoea. Complications include inflammation of the internal genital organs and may have serious consequences especially for women, including infertility. It is important that investigation of genito-urinary disease should include a search for this organism. In the process of birth, babies can receive an infection leading to pneumonia or more commonly conjunctivitis.

Sexually transmitted infections caused by viruses are in the industrialised countries now more commonly reported than the classic bacterial infections. Genital herpes has been rising more steeply in reported incidence than any other notifiable sexually transmitted disease, the high reporting rate being perhaps due to its known association with carcinoma of the cervix and transmission to the newborn. Genital warts, also of viral origin, have become extremely common, and treatment is so ineffective that a great deal of medical time is taken up with trying to deal with them.

Cytomegalovirus

There are three other virus infections of major significance. The first is infection by the cytomegalovirus, which is commonly spread by sexual intercourse among young adults in developed countries and is responsible for a substantial proportion of congenital birth defects such as deafness, mental retardation and severe damage to the internal organs. There are about 3000 new congenital infections each year in Britain, 300 of which result in subsequent handicap. Cytomegalovirus is excreted in the urine of about 3% of apparently healthy pregnant women and by about 1% of newborn babies, most of whom show no effects of harm. However, this virus is now a more frequent cause of congenital mental retardation than rubella. It is one of the (rare) causes of viral hepatitis.

Hepatitis B

Hepatitis B is caused by a highly infectious and sturdy virus carried particularly in blood but also in any other of the body's fluids, including saliva, vaginal secretions, semen, menses, tears and vomit. Any of these fluids can transmit the disease from one person to another, usually through the skin or mucous membranes.

The illness caused by the hepatitis B virus results from inflammation of the liver, and the symptoms and signs are very similar to those of hepatitis A. More than half of the infections result in minor illness for which medical attention is unlikely to be sought. But it can lead to two serious complications. One is that around one in ten of those who recover from the acute illness can become carriers, and continue to transmit the disease for life without themselves feeling ill in any way. The other is that resulting longstanding inflammation of the liver tissue can progress to cancer, and in some places in the world primary liver cancer is one of the commonest cancers of all, especially among men. In Taiwan, for example, it represents nearly a quarter of all cancers, and about 80% are caused by the hepatitis B virus.

Accordingly, the vast majority of those who are infectious do not know that they are, either because their illness has been mild or because they are carriers without symptoms.

There are an enormous number of carriers in the world: the true number cannot possibly be known, but an informed estimate is at least 200 million, or in the order of 5% of the entire global population. Carriers are very commonly identified in parts of tropical Africa and South-East Asia (10–20% of the population), but are comparatively rare in northern Europe, North America and Australasia (averaging up to 1%).

Interest in what was known as serum hepatitis was sharply awakened in 1942, when several thousands of American military personnel developed jaundice after being immunised against yellow fever. Continuing research, bolstered by re-examination of several earlier studies, showed that a proportion of people must be carrying something in their blood which, when injected into other people by blood transfusion or via serum in a vaccine, caused hepatitis. But it was a completely unrelated research programme which uncovered the hepatitis B virus.

A geneticist, B. S. Blumberg, was examining genetic disturbances in the proteins of human serum, and during a study of racial differences found that serum from an Australian aborigine reacted in a unique way with the serum from a patient who had been given many blood transfusions. He assumed that the blood from Australian aborigines must contain a characteristic protein, and called it 'Australia antigen', but it soon became clear that this antigen had nothing at all to do with race. Antibodies to it could be found in the blood of many hospital patients in the United States, and the electron microscope showed that in the same blood were particles ('Dane particles')

Figure 52   Structure of hepatitis B virus, now recognised as being an important blood-borne disease and a prime cause of liver cancer.

Structure of Hepatitis B Virus

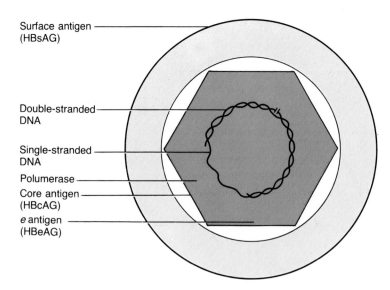

Surface antigen (HBsAG)

Double-stranded DNA

Single-stranded DNA

Polumerase

Core antigen (HBcAG)

e antigen (HBeAG)

with the characteristics of a virus.

The hepatitis B virus is a complicated structure. It is a DNA virus, with integration of the virus DNA with the cell DNA of the host being the reason for the life-long effects of infection. The central core of the virus carries the infection, the antigen being known as 'hepatitis B core antigen', or HBcAg. On the surface of the virus is the antigen first identified as the Australia antigen, now known as 'hepatitis B surface antigen', or HBsAg. Diagnosis of the disease or of the carrier state depends on identification in the blood of 'markers', which are various components of the antigen-antibody system, including HBsAg, the antibody to the surface antigen (anti-HBs), and the antibody to the core antigen (anti-HBc).

Hepatitis B is transmitted by close personal contact including sexual relationships; the sexually promiscuous, therefore, especially male homosexuals, are at particularly high risk of contracting the disease. Anything that can inoculate minute amounts of blood can transmit the disease, including dental, surgical and nursing procedures, drug abuse using injections, tattooing, ear piercing and acupuncture. Accidental inoculation can occur by way of what is known in evocative medical jargon as 'needle-stick injury'. The virus is so infective that there is an up to 40% chance of contracting the disease following accidental exposure to the blood of a patient with

acute hepatitis or carrying the surface antigen, with the analogous risk for the AIDS virus being less than 1%.

Repeated investigations of medical and dental personnel have shown that both the rate of infection with the virus, and the prevalence in the blood of markers showing previous infection, are several times above the population average, with large variations from country to country. An illustrative case occurred in New South Wales, where an outbreak of hepatitis B among health care workers was traced to the victim of a motorcycle crash who was incubating the disease. An ambulance officer cut his hands on glass at the scene of the accident; a surgeon splashed blood into his eye during the operation; two intensive care nurses spilt dialysis fluid on to cut hands; an operating theatre aide cut a hand on the glass of a broken suction bottle; and an intensive care nurse changed a bloodstained bandage with cuts on his hands. All developed the disease.

The risk faced by medical and dental personnel in dealing with the infected, with the potentially infected and with carriers is such that special measures such as immunisation now need to be taken for their protection, and this is a matter discussed in more detail in the next chapter.

Mothers who are carriers can transmit the infection to their babies at around the time of birth, and this appears to be the most important way the

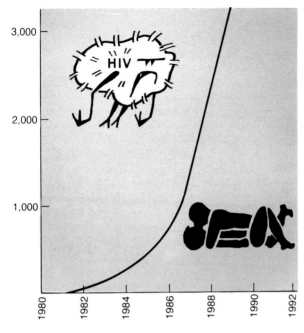

AIDS : estimated new cases in Britain

Figure 53   The incidence of AIDS is rising steeply and, because of the long period between infection and the onset of the disease, control measures are inevitably delayed in their effect.

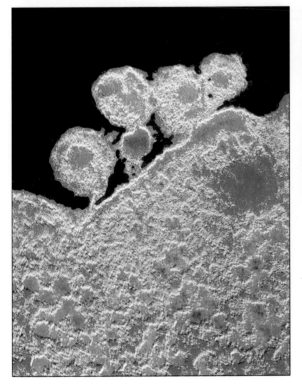

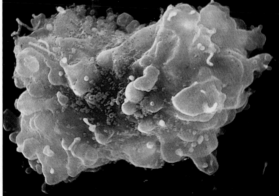

Figure 54   The Human Immunodeficiency Virus (HIV) infects the T4 lymphocyte, where the viral RNA is permanently inserted into the cell DNA. Copies of the virus are produced and the infectious particles are expressed into the circulating blood

(a) False-colour transmission electron micrograph of HIV particles emerging from T4 lymphocyte; (magnification × 105,000)

(b) Scanning electron micrograph of T4 cell with (blue) virus particles on cell surface disease is transmitted in South-East Asia. The risk of infection is greatest if the mother has a history of transmission to previous children, and has a high titre of hepatitis B surface antigen (HBsAg) and/or e antigen.

As the disease is carried in the blood, there is natural concern that blood transmitted from person to person by the bites and stings of arthropods and animals could be a route of transmission, but there is only conflicting and doubtful evidence that the virus multiplies within the bodies of insects. However, it is theoretically possible for the biting parts to transmit the virus mechanically.

Laboratory work on hepatitis A and hepatitis B has led to the discovery that there are other forms of hepatitis caused by neither of these two viruses nor any other identifiable organism, and these are called non-A, and non-B hepatitis. In some countries these are the commonest forms of hepatitis to follow the transfusion of blood. Cancer of the liver can be a consequence of infection by the non-A, non-B viruses.

Human immunodeficiency virus (HIV)

The third of these three viral contact diseases is now the best known among the general public in the developed world, because of its lethal nature and the unprecedented public educational measures being employed in some countries to try to control its escalating incidence. HIV is, of course, the causative organism of the acquired immune deficiency syndrome, universally known as AIDS, to which we have already referred in the context of diseases of the body's immune system.

The syndrome, initially identified as rare forms of pneumonia and skin cancer in patients with deficiencies in their immune systems, was first reported in the United States in late 1981, although it is now suspected from retrospective analysis (in some cases of the body tissues of people who died mysteriously, stored for later detective work) that a few people had suffered the disease many years before in the United States, the Caribbean and Africa. During the early stages of its spread in developed countries, it appeared almost exclusively in the homosexual and intravenous drug-using populations, and heterosexual transmission was relatively uncommon. However, in places such as equatorial Africa, the disease is transmitted mainly by heterosexual

contact. Because of its recent recognition, the epidemiology of AIDS is still far from being completely understood, and there are many aspects of its spread which will no doubt be clarified in the future.

AIDS is caused by a virus which has gone through a few name changes but which is now referred to as the human immunodeficiency virus, or HIV. It has been isolated from several of the body's secretions, but evidence relating to transmission has implicated mainly blood, semen and the vaginal secretions. It employs the same blood-to-blood routes of transmission as the virus of hepatitis B, being transmitted by anal and vaginal intercourse, and by direct transmission in contaminated blood by way of infected needles (usually among drug-using groups) and blood and some blood products. It can also be passed by an infected mother to her child before birth.

It is not, as viruses go, particularly infectious, far less infectious than that of hepatitis B. Long-term partners of those with the disease, for example, have failed to contract it themselves. No evidence exists that the infection can be transmitted by casual contact of the sort that occurs during day-to-day household activities, and even among the thousands of health workers caring for AIDS patients only a handful have been infected. The risk of acquiring infection after being accidentally pricked with an infected needle is less than 1%, compared for example to at least a 20% risk which exists after being pricked with an infected needle used while caring for a patient with hepatitis B.

When HIV penetrates a cell in the human body, an enzyme (characteristic of a 'retrovirus') converts RNA in the virus into DNA, which then becomes integrated into the DNA of the new host cell. Thus, when the host cells reproduce, they carry the genes of the virus with them. This results in an infection which lasts for life.

The incidence of AIDS is increasing at epidemic rates in the developed countries, and in the developing countries – whose official position had in a few cases been that the disease was unknown – the numbers are also rising rapidly as the accuracy of reporting improves.

In the UK by the end of September 1988, 1794 cases of AIDS had been reported (the disease is not an officially notifiable one). In the United States 70702 cases had been reported by mid-August. In the developed world, unless present trends can be substantially changed, AIDS will by the end of this century have overtaken road accidents as a cause of death, and be the main single killer of young men.

A long period usually exists between infection by HIV and the occurrence of the full syndrome, and it is still not known what proportion of those now infected will become ill later; in Europe, some half a million people were estimated to be infected by late 1987, and between 25,000 and 30,000 cases of AIDS were estimated by the WHO to be likely to have occurred by the end of 1988. In the United States, experts believe that by 1991 there will have been a cumulative total of 270,000 cases of AIDS in that country, with 179,000 deaths. As to the total of the HIV-infected people in the world, the late-1987 estimate of the WHO of 50–100 million by 1991 will be conservative if HIV penetrates and spreads through South America and Asia. Because of the long incubation period of the disease, most of the people who will develop AIDS between now and 1991 are already infected, and the late-1987 estimate of the WHO was for between half a million and three million new cases of the syndrome to emerge by 1991.

Hospital infection

While not all hospital-acquired infections (sometimes known, especially in the United States, as 'nosocomial' infections) occur as a result of transmission by direct contact, so many of them do that it is appropriate to discuss them in this section.

Hospitals developed as places where the sick could be treated and subjected to scholarly investigation while grouped together, a fine intention, but one which did not work out as envisaged because the patients and staff infected each other to an extent that the places of supposed healing became death traps. The findings of Semmelweiss on the transmission of puerperal fever, and the slow development of antiseptic and aseptic surgical techniques, gradually made treatment in hospitals less lethal, and with the development of antibiotic drugs it was thought that the problem of hospital infection was beaten for ever. Again, however, things did not work out as expected, and hospitals became breeding grounds for new strains of bacteria which were just as virulent as their forebears but resistant to the measures and chemicals used to kill them. The battle against infection in hospitals is a never-ending one, and will remain so as long as sick, vulnerable and infected people are treated within them.

In Britain, up to 16% of patients acquire new infections while in hospital. Most, fortunately, are not very serious, but they can be so for some particular patients. People most at risk of becoming infected are those whose general defences are down as a result of age, illness or treatment (such as that for cancer), and those whose skin and membrane barriers have been breached by injury or some sort of medical procedure (such as in immuno-suppression therapy following transplantation of an organ).

The four infections most commonly acquired in hospital are those of wounds inflicted by surgery, of the urinary tract, of the lower respiratory tract, and of the skin (in the form of ulcers and sores).

The type of surgical wound that presents the greatest risk of infection involves sites where pathogens are normally to be found, such as in the bowel. Appendicectomy is a common example. Naturally, surgery on already infected sites (such as abscesses or motor vehicle injuries) carries a special risk of additional infection.

Urinary tract infections probably account for at least one-quarter of hospital-acquired infections, the responsible micro-organisms usually coming from the patient's own faecal flora. The infection is commonly transmitted during a procedure such as catheterisation of the bladder.

Lower respiratory tract infections are relatively common in the elderly, especially those who have to lie in bed and who have a pre-existing chest problem or are heavy smokers.

The organisms causing hospital infections include the streptococci and staphylococci and others that are commonly encountered elsewhere. Many infections are from the patients' own flora, and can be carried on the hands of attendants to other patients.

The speed and extent of spread of an infection depends a great deal on the extent to which the organism is resistant to antibiotics. Streptococci almost always respond to penicillin, but many other bacteria are resistant to a wide variety of antibiotics. The pattern of resistance may, in fact, help in determining the source of the outbreak.

As we have suggested above, the control of hospital infection is now is its own right a matter of major endeavour, and a special section is allotted to the subject in the next chapter.

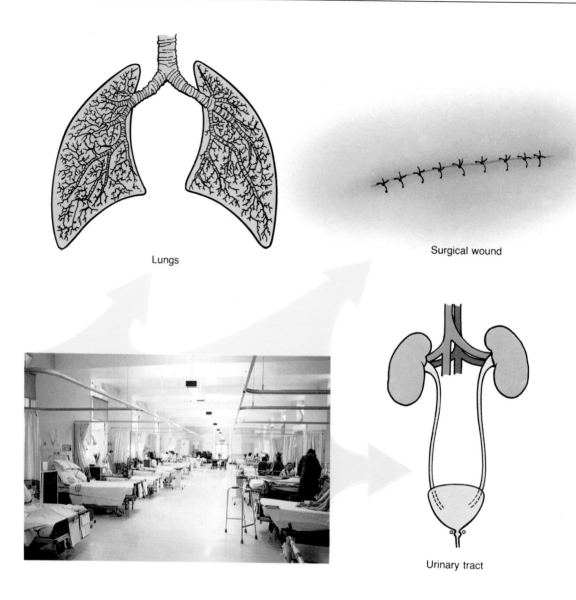

Lungs

Surgical wound

Urinary tract

Figure 55   The most common hospital infections are those following surgery, those of the urinary and respiratory systems, and those of the skin.

ARTHROPODS AS VECTORS

Scores of different types of living creatures play a part in the transmission of infectious disease from man to man and from animal to man. Numerically, most of the world's diseases are carried by arthropods (insects and their close relatives).

In most cases, the infection is introduced into the tissues by bites or stings, although transmission may also be mechanical, as on the feet of flies, beetles and cockroaches.

Arthropod means 'jointed leg', and these creatures are all characterised by an external skeleton and jointed appendages including legs, mouth parts and antennae. The total number of them is vast, but only a few transmit communicable disease to man. Among those that do are mosquitoes, ticks, lice, mites, fleas and flies. Some of them, such as the scabies mite, are external parasites of man but not normally vectors of disease.

Fortunately, all the diseases spread in this way are now rare in developed countries in the temperate climates of the world. However, among them are the major epidemic diseases of malaria, plague and typhus, and these were all once widespread in Europe, including Britain; while conditions at present would prevent their re-emergence, the necessary biological mechanisms and vectors all still exist to take advantage of any fundamental breakdown in public order. In other parts of the world the protozoal disease malaria is still one of the very commonest serious illnesses. Adding to the toll, the number of viruses which are now known to be carried by arthropods and rodents is nearly 500, some 97 of which are pathogenic for man.

Many of the diseases transmitted to humans by arthropods are not really diseases of man at all but 'zoonoses', being primarily diseases of animals. The species from which the arthropod vector picks up the organism is usually the reservoir of the disease. In most cases there is a complicated interaction between the micro-organism, the arthropod vector, the vertebrate or invertebrate host, man, and the environment, and this will determine the speed and ferocity of spread of the disease.

What usually happens is that an arthropod feeds on an infected host (man or otherwise), becomes infected itself, and after a variable period during which the organism develops and/or multiplies within it, transmits it to another vertebrate while feeding on its blood. This whole process is a biological rather than a mechanical one. However, it is also possible to transmit organisms purely mechanically, with the arthropod carrying what are customarily in this case viruses on the mouth parts from one animal to another as a 'flying pin', as it is sometimes known. Another mechanical method is used by some lice and fleas, which release the infecting organisms in faeces while they are feeding, with the result that the infection is passed through the skin by the itching, scratching host. Flies can carry pathogenic organisms – such as those causing typhoid and dysentery – on their feet from faeces to food.

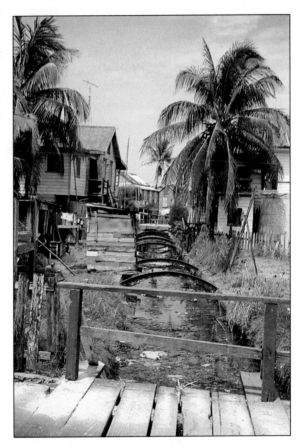

Figure 56 Belize City, Central America. Malaria may be prevalent wherever mosquitos can breed in marshy or stagnant areas, and control of the disease depends in part on modification of the environment to eliminate such breeding grounds.

Mosquitoes and malaria

Mosquitoes, the first example of a few vectors whose activities we will examine in more detail, spread serious life-threatening and incapacitating diseases to millions of people all around the world every year. These include malaria and a wide variety of arthropod-borne viruses (arboviruses) such as dengue and yellow fever, plus many more which are often denominated by the name of the region in which the condition is prevalent: Japanese encephalitis, California encephalitis, Murray Valley encephalitis, Rift Valley fever, St Louis encephalitis and many others.

Malaria is the commonest arthropod-borne disease to be seen in Britain because it is commonly imported, but others are rare. (The life cycle of the malaria parasite, and its relationship to the anopheles mosquito, is described in the section on the protozoa in Chapter 4.) Each year the number of cases officially reported in the UK ranges between about 1,500 and 2,200, with no consistent trend being revealed, with deaths averaging between six and seven a year.

The disease has been known for centuries, and Hippocrates described what appear to be the different forms of malaria in his work, *Epidemics*. It was endemic in the Mediterranean basin until quite recently, and it is one of those diseases which some suppose to have contributed to the decline of civilisations including ancient Greece and the Roman Empire. Indeed, malaria was a very common affliction in the marshy areas round Rome, and the Roman army was under orders to avoid such areas for fear of fever. In Britain, where it was known as the 'ague', malaria was endemic in marshy parts of the country until less than 100 years ago: the Fens and the Thames Estuary were the areas most affected. Quinine was recognised as a remedy in Italy and the Spanish American colonies by 1650, but Oliver Cromwell banned the importation to Protestant England of a medicine known as 'Jesuits' power' and, for his pains, died a little later from 'the ague'. Mosquitoes capable of transmitting malaria still exist in Britain, and there are people with malarial parasites in their blood, but the number of the latter is too small, and the average temperatures now too low for development of the sporozoites in the mosquitoes, to allow an endemic situation ever to be likely again.

As noted in the section on the protozoa, Patrick Manson, the pioneer in tropical medicine, discovered the role of the mosquito in transmitting filariasis in 1877, and this led to suggestions that the mosquito could also be transmitting yellow fever. In 1882 these suggestions flowed on to malaria, and preliminary suggestions on controlling the spread by means of mosquito netting and the drainage of swamps and pools were first put forward. The actual malaria parasite was first seen in human blood in 1880 by the French surgeon Laveran, and his speculations on the role of mosquitoes in marshy areas drew the attention of a strong team of scientists in Rome, where the disease appeared in regular waves. A Scottish physician and protégé of Manson, Ronald Ross, worked out the life cycle of the malaria parasite and the part played by the mosquito in transmitting the disease while working in the Indian Medical Service, meticulous work for which he received a Nobel Prize, but his discoveries were matched almost simultaneously by other workers in Rome and the United States.

Discovery of the role of the mosquito pointed the way to control, but it was to take the priorities of war to stimulate the development of truly effective countermeasures. Soldiers in the second world war were falling victim to the disease in some areas as often as to the battle. During the march of the British and United States armies up through Sicily and southern Italy, the advance was severely retarded by rain, mud and malaria; the equivalent of two infantry divisions were incapacitated by malaria, although fortunately not fatally. In the Pacific in the second world war and the Korean war, the American troops suffered terribly from malaria, and the same happened during and after the war in Vietnam. The development of effective methods of mosquito control in 1940–45 led to huge improvements in Europe by 1960, and it became envisaged by WHO planners that the worldwide elimination of the disease was a practical possibility. Unfortunately, as will be seen in Chapter 9, that was an impossible dream, but malaria has indeed been banished from great areas where once it ran rife.

The arboviruses: yellow fever and dengue

Much attention is currently being paid to the role of arthropods in transmitting viral diseases, caused by the so-called arboviruses. Among those that are transmitted by mosquitoes, the WHO is focusing its attention particularly on the three important diseases, yellow fever, dengue fever, and Rift Valley fever, all of which are notable because of their ability to cause large and often unpredicted epidemic outbreaks. These all fall into the group of 'haemorrhagic fevers', which have similar clinical characteristics but different epidemiological features. Some, like yellow fever, have been known for centuries, whereas the majority have emerged more recently either because they have a newly-developed potential for spreading or because they have only just been recognised at all. The total number of affected people is comparatively small, but the diseases are troubling to communities and public health administrations because the death rate from each one is high, and all are unusually difficult to treat and to prevent.

Typically, the patient feels ill with flu-like symptoms about a week after being bitten, and if the disease progresses tiny bleeding points appear under the skin and mucous membranes. Bleeding may also occur internally. In the very worst cases the patient collapses into shock, which may be irreversible. Yellow fever is typically accompanied by the jaundice which gives it its name.

Yellow fever is the only one of this group of diseases to have been recognised for long enough to have a history, and an interesting history it is too. It was one of the major epidemic scourges of Europe and the New World from the mid-sixteenth century until the beginning of the twentieth – 60,000 people died in Spain alone in 1800. Yet within 20 years of the discovery in 1901 that it was caused by something in the blood and carried by a mosquito, concentrated and intensive control measures directed specifically towards the mode of transmission of the disease had eliminated it from the United States, Central America and the Caribbean, and most of South America.

The origin of yellow fever was probably in west Africa, and this was also the origin of the slaves with whom the disease travelled to the New World. The female of the mosquito species *Aëdes aegypti* developed a preference for depositing her eggs in man-made water containers, and it was the drinking water casks of the slave ships which carried the larvae to the new colonies. It was first recognised in Mexico in 1648, from where it surged down the Spanish Main and caused havoc among the marauding Spanish and English soldiers and buccaneers. It curved through the Caribbean chain of islands, where the largely immune African slaves were little affected, and up the great Amazon and Mississippi rivers. From the New World it bounced back to the Old, along with the returning sailors, soldiers and explorers.

Epidemics occurred up and down the east coast of the north American continent throughout the seventeenth, eighteenth and nineteenth centuries, provoking great controversy between the anticontagionists, who believed that atmospheric and miasmic influences should be countered by improvements in cleanliness and sanitation, and the contagionists, who believed that the disease was being imported and that quarantine restrictions should be applied. To some extent, of course, the efforts of both sides contributed to the eventual control of the disease. In hindsight, it is easy to point to lucky guesses and attribute to their originators an unwarranted degree of scientific insight, but it is worth recording that at the height of a dreadful epidemic in Philadelphia, while cannon were being shot off in the streets and people were wearing ropes of garlic and tar round their necks as antidotes, an anonymous correspondent wrote to the paper pointing out the great increase in 'poisonous' mosquitoes during the rain, and suggested that their breeding be stopped by putting oil on the surface of water tubs. Meanwhile, across the Atlantic, exploration of west Africa was becoming a suicidal activity for Europeans, with yellow fever joining other fatal maladies to give the region its reputation as 'the white man's grave'.

By the end of the last century yellow fever was having such an influence on the turn of great international affairs that research on it had become a highly serious matter. The trigger that fired the gun that solved the problem was the Spanish-American war of 1898 and the subsequent occupation of Cuba by American troops, among whom an appalling toll was taken by the disease. A Cuban physician had, since 1881, been convinced that mosquitoes bore the disease to man, and his work was the basis on which a US Army board started its own investigations. The board was headed by Major Walter Reed, and it was his team, aided by Major William Gorgas (to achieve fame by wiping out yellow fever and malaria during the building of the canal across Panama a few years later), that finally identified the responsible mosquito, the infectious nature of the blood in the mosquito and in man, and the timing of the cycle of infectivity. This was enough virtually to eliminate yellow fever as a serious problem in Cuba within a single year (1901–02), long before it was proved in 1929 that a virus was the responsible organism.

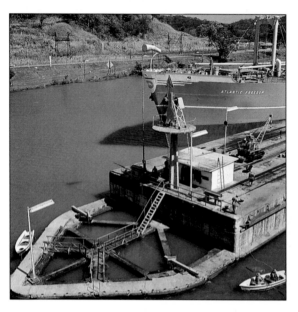

Figure 57   The extraordinary achievement of the building of the Panama Canal was not only one of engineering but also of infection control, as yellow fever and malaria had to be eliminated before the canal could be completed.

It took brave men to do this research. One member of the Reed board died, and at a time when the death rate approached 85% three young American soldiers volunteered as human guinea pigs (and survived). In establishing the viral cause of the disease a group of American and English scientists, financed by the Rockefeller Foundation, were working with monkeys in west Africa when one of the English scientists became infected and died. Two Japanese scientists joined this group, one of them being a prominent bacteriologist at the Rockefeller Institute, and both of them perished as well. Soon, however, a vaccine was developed and the disease ceased to present such a dreadful threat.

Yellow fever is still endemic in tropical regions of the Americas and Africa, but not Asia. It is primarily a disease of monkeys, transmitted by the mosquito *Aëdes aegypti* from monkeys to monkeys and from monkeys to man ('jungle yellow fever'), and, once well established, from man to man ('urban yellow fever'). Outbreaks tend to occur in particular areas after long periods; there were outbreaks in Colombia and Trinidad in 1978–79 after more than 19 years free from the fever, and in Bolivia after 30 years.

The *Aëdes* mosquito is distributed very widely in the world, including Europe and Asia, where yellow fever has not been seen, and strenuous efforts are necessary to prevent the present boundaries extending. Urban yellow fever can be kept under control, but because the disease will inevitably continue to circulate among monkeys in the jungle, it will always be impossible to eliminate jungle yellow fever and thus eradicate the disease as a whole.

Dengue haemorrhagic fever is caused by the group of dengue viruses, another group of the mosquito-borne arboviruses. The ubiquitous mosquito *Aëdes aegypti* is again the main vector, being a domestic mosquito that likes to feed on human blood.

The term 'dengue' includes the common and relatively mild classical dengue, also known as 'breakbone fever' because of the pain in the spine and joints it causes, as well as the rarer haemorrhagic fever, which causes shock and a high mortality rate, particularly among the young. Unusually, animals play virtually no part in the circulation of the disease. The viruses have been prevalent in tropical Africa and the Americas for years, and outbreaks have also been identified in the Mediterranean basin, South-East Asia and the western Pacific. The fullblown fever has become one of the most important causes of morbidity and mortality among children in South-East Asia, and it is currently prevalent throughout that region, the western Pacific, India and the Caribbean. In 1981, dengue haemorrhagic fever killed 158 people in Cuba, about two-thirds of them being children under 15.

Sandflies of the genus *Phlebotomus* are the vectors for the leishmaniases in the Old World, as we noted earlier when discussing the protozoal diseases. With their relations in the New World, about 70 species of sandfly spread this group of diseases, some of which can be unpleasant souvenirs of a Mediterranean holiday. They breed in rich, damp soil, and pick up the parasites from the reservoirs, which are dogs, rats and small wild mammals.

Ticks

Ticks, like mosquitoes, spread arboviruses which cause various kinds of haemorrhagic fever found in eastern Europe, the USSR and India. In addition, they carry many of the rickettsial micro-organisms, causing a group of diseases which are clinically very similar and distributed throughout the world. These include scrub typhus (tsutsugamushi disease, also carried by mites), Rocky Mountain spotted fever, and the related Q ('Query') fever. These illnesses vary greatly in their lethal potential for man, who becomes quite accidentally involved in the parasitic relationship between organism, tick, and the various animals – including dogs, cats, rats, rabbits and bandicoots – on which the tick depends for its blood meals.

Of interest because of recent sporadic cases in the UK and Ireland is Lyme disease, named after a district in Connecticut which is one of many areas where it is endemic. It is caused by a spirochaete, *Borrelia burgdorferi*, with small mammals serving as reservoirs and transmission being through the bites of ticks. Patients suffer recurrent disabling and sometimes destructive attacks of arthritis of the large joints, and may also suffer from inflammation of the brain and nervous system. In 1986 there were 68 cases of Lyme disease in the UK and Ireland, and in some areas around two-thirds of deer, the suspected reservoir, were found to be infected with the spirochaete.

Lice

It is not the tick but the humble human body louse, *Pediculus humanus*, which is responsible for spreading the most famous of the rickettsial diseases, epidemic typhus, and is thus another tiny creature which has played a part in the history of mankind. Classic epidemic typhus is a disease which is uniquely human, and has frequently occurred in major pandemic form, generally in association with war, famine and poverty. It is what we usually mean when we refer to 'typhus', as opposed to the rickettsial diseases spread by ticks and mites, and it still exists in endemic form in Asia, Africa and mountainous parts of Central and South America. The disease is manifest by fever, prostration, body pains and a rash; the fatality rate varies from 10–40%, increasing with age. Man is infected by scratching faeces or crushed lice into

the itchy bites; he, in turn, infects lice when they feed on his blood. The lice invariably die within two weeks of infection, which has led historians of biology to conclude that the louse is a new host for the organisms in the evolutionary sense, having long beforehand lived as a parasite of man without either participant in the relationship getting typhus fever.

The disease takes its worst form in epidemics during the sort of social upheaval that occurs during war; in quieter times, although conditions still may encourage body lice to live on man, the endemic form gives rise to a comparatively mild illness.

From the fifteenth to the nineteenth century, typhus took a shocking toll of lives in armies, prisons and ships. Military doctors played a tremendous part in recognising the connection between dirt and the disease, with Sir John Pringle in the army and James Lind in the Royal Navy doing a huge amount to improve conditions of

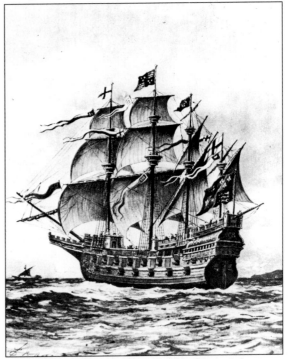

Figure 58 Infectious disease has always taken a terrible toll among fighting men, and war has often been a stimulus to infection control measures. In the Royal Navy, infection aboard ship could decimate the crew, and naval doctors were pioneers in ensuring a high standard of hygiene for the prevention of disease.

hygiene in the British armed forces in the eighteenth century. However, while on the western front of the first world war typhus was kept under remarkable control, it raged over eastern Europe and, indeed, influenced the course of the Russian Revolution in 1917, when millions in that country died from its ravages. Although thousands of civilians suffered from typhus in North Africa during the second world war, only a handful of troops were infected, because of sanitary measures and the use of an effective vaccine. The remarkable elimination of typhus from Naples after the war is described when control measures are examined in more detail later.

Fleas

Fleas we have mentioned earlier in the context of bubonic plague, when describing the place of this disease in the history of the great epidemic infections. Plague is a disease specifically of rats and their fleas, which transmit the disease to other animals, including man. It causes swelling of the lymph nodes (the 'buboes' of bubonic plague), and in a severe form, pneumonia. Over vast areas of the globe wild rodents with plague still roam, and outbreaks of human plague have recently occurred in several countries in Africa, Burma and Vietnam. Some dozens of cases still occur each year in the United States. Untreated, the death rate is about 50% but modern therapy has markedly reduced this.

Flies

Flies, as every child is taught at school, spread disease, usually by carrying the organisms responsible for intestinal illnesses from faeces to food. This a fly does by carrying faecal material on its legs, by regurgitating the contents of its stomach on its food in order to liquefy it, and by defaecating on its food.

In Africa, the tsetse fly carries the protozoa responsible for trypanosomiasis, or sleeping sickness, a name which probably sprang from a description of the disease given by John Atkins, an English naval surgeon, who wrote of 'somnolence' among the local population and a high death rate. Although confined to tropical Africa, the disease is still not under control, and in some endemic regions up to 30% of the population have been infected.

DISEASES OF ANIMALS AND MAN

Animals can pass diseases to man through all the pathways described above: by the airborne route, by ingestion of faecal matter or inhalation of dried faeces, by direct contact with the animal's skin or saliva as it bites or licks, and by way of an intermediate vector such as a mosquito. In addition, man may become infected through ingestion of infected animal products such as meat and milk. Generally, the diseases are zoonoses, conditions which are essentially diseases of vertebrate animals, and if the routes of transmission are understood then the diseases are open to control.

Infected food and milk

In the earlier section on food poisoning, we described how infections in animals can be passed to man as a result of improper preparation of food from animal products, with salmonellosis in poultry and campylobacter infections being perhaps the most important examples. Milk, if not pasteurised, can be the vehicle for carrying several zoonoses to man, including the bovine type of tuberculosis, brucellosis and toxoplasmosis.

Brucellosis is an infection of the genital and urinary tracts of cattle, goats, sheep, pigs and dogs by various species of the *Brucella* bacterium. It causes abortion in animals, and the organisms abound in any of the proceeds of abortion and subsequent discharges, and settle in the uterus, udder and associated lymph glands. They may then be excreted in the milk, and humans are infected when they consume milk or milk products which are thus contaminated. Farm workers can also become infected by direct contact with the infected animal's genital tract during, for example, the process of birth or abortion.

Brucellosis represented a serious threat to food supplies and animal health until well after the second world war, when the WHO and the Food and Agriculture Organisation combined to combat it. While the disease is now rare in Britain, North America and Australasia, it still occurs in many other countries of the world, causing perhaps more human illness than any other animal disease.

It has existed for centuries in the Mediterranean basin, where fresh milk, cheese and yogurt are especially popular, and one of its many synonyms is Mediterranean fever. Others are Malta fever, Cyprus fever, Gibraltar fever and undulant fever (because the temperature of a sufferer goes up and down). Australian-born British army surgeon David Bruce found the cause of the human disease during a series of studies in Malta during the first years of this century, and when British soldiers were forbidden to drink goats' milk, the incidence of brucellosis among them decreased almost to zero.

The human illness is a vague and prolonged one, with a swinging fever, aches and pains, loss of appetite and weight. Recovery normally occurs by itself, which is fortunate because of the lack of response of the organism to antibiotics, but in a few cases the disease causes complications in the bones and nervous system. Prevention is by pasteurisation of milk and through more general knowledge of the risks of eating and drinking milk products in countries where the disease is prevalent. In Britain and similar countries infected herds are slaughtered.

Pets

Because an animal is a favoured member of a human household is no guarantee that it is free from a zoonosis which can be transmitted to its fond owners. Examples we described in Chapter 4 were: toxoplasmosis, a protozoal disease of cats, which if contracted by a pregnant woman can result in damage to the foetus; and hydatid disease, a tapeworm infestation of dogs which can give rise to dangerous cysts in man. There are many others, and children are especially vulnerable because of the closely affectionate relationship they often have with their pets. Below, therefore, we outline the characteristics of a few of the more important zoonoses, ones which may be encountered in northern Europe, and more are listed in Appendix B.

A disease of probably worldwide distribution but which has aroused particular interest in Britain and the United States is toxocariasis, which causes a long lasting but usually mild illness in young children as larvae of the *Toxocara* roundworm move throughout the body tissues. The reservoir of the disease is in cats of all ages, and dogs, especially puppies. Children acquire it by ingesting soil which has been contaminated by the animal faeces. Such contamination should be avoided around houses and children's play areas; sand pits,

unfortunately, are attractive places for cats to defaecate. To prevent infection, dogs and cats can be regularly dewormed. Children, especially, should be encouraged to avoid letting pets lick their faces, and in general hands should be thoroughly washed after playing outside and with pet animals. Drug treatment for the infected children is available, but effectiveness is poor.

In tropical areas, dogs and cats can act as reservoirs for a very wide range of other protozoal and helminthic diseases, including schistosomiasis, hookworm disease and sleeping sickness. They can also transmit mycoses to man, such as the familiar tinea. 'Cat- scratch fever' is a mild and rare illness of obvious direct cause, but the organism is so far unidentified. All scratches from cats (and other animals) should be very thoroughly washed.

An important bacterial illness which is carried by pets, and especially puppies and kittens, is *Campylobacter* diarrhoea, which can be serious in young children. They should never, therefore, be allowed to play with pets which themselves have any signs of diarrhoea, and, again, washing the hands after playing with animals is a sound precaution in any event.

Leptospirosis is caused by a type of spirochaete which survives in water and wet soil, settles in animal kidneys and is excreted in the urine. It has several other names depending on its manifestation. It is a worldwide hazard to all who deal closely with pets as well as domestic and wild animals, and to those who work in farms (it is perhaps the commonest occupational disease of all in New Zealand), paddies, sewers and mines. The disease is not usually very serious, with many vague symptoms including fever, headache, vomiting and a rash. Transmission is through direct contact by human skin or mucous membranes with the urine of infected animals, or with soil, water or vegetation contaminated by urine.

There are scores of varieties of the organism, but the main ones fall into three groups. The first is *Leptospira icterohaemorrhagiae*, for which rats are the best-known reservoir; Weil's disease is a common name, an occupational hazard of sewer workers which is characterised by jaundice. *Leptospira hebdomadis*, carried by cattle and small wild animals such as field mice, voles and hedgehogs, poses a threat to farm workers. In pets, *Leptospira canicola* is carried by dogs in particular, as well as by horses and a number of farm animals.

The human disease is sometimes known as 'canicola fever', and can be serious enough to cause meningitis in children playing with infected puppies.

Psittacosis, caused by *Chlamydia psittaci*, is a disease of birds such as parrots and budgerigars, and man becomes infected by way of direct contact by inhaling dust which has been infected by droppings. Ornithosis is a similar chlamydial disease carried by other types of bird. It occurs world wide, and a few hundred cases occur in Britain each year. The illness affects the respiratory tract and may progress to pneumonia. In sheep, the same organism causes abortion, stillbirth and sickly lambs, and in a few cases pregnant women attending infected ewes during the lambing season have themselves become infected, with severe illness and abortion being among the outcomes.

The more unusual the pet, the greater the risk that it may be carrying an unexpected disease. For those few readers who may be contemplating keeping such a creature, it may be worth citing as an example the fact that alligators are common carriers of salmonella.

Rabies

Perhaps the most feared zoonosis of all, one that is carried by dogs, cats and many other domestic and wild mammals, is the viral disease rabies. The saliva from a rabid animal, loaded with the rabies virus, is punched through the skin by a bite (in Europe, most commonly from a dog) or, very rarely, a scratch. A feeling of apprehension leads on to fever and malaise, then paralysis which often starts in the neck muscles and gives difficulty swallowing (including water; hence the old name, 'hydrophobia'). The illness, which is almost invariably fatal, only lasts from two to six days.

Rabies is fortunately uncommon in man. Wild carnivores are the main transmitters of wildlife rabies, and large populations of the animals, together with a long incubation period, allow the disease to remain endemic (enzootic, strictly speaking) even though the host in each case will inevitably die. In Europe the red fox is the main carrier, with foxes, skunks and raccoons being of importance in the United States. A small Indian mongoose has recently been introduced into the Caribbean, and is propagating the disease to the accompaniment of some alarm, because it attacks domestic animals and man. Bats are carriers in the Americas and especially in Central and South America, where vampire bats exact a terrible toll among domestic cattle.

Among areas at present reported to be free from rabies in the animal kingdom are Australia, New Zealand, the Malaysian peninsula, Japan, Hawaii, Taiwan and other Pacific islands, the United Kingdom, Ireland, Spain, Portugal, mainland Norway, Sweden, and some parts of the West Indies and Atlantic islands. All such places impose demanding restrictions on the importation of domestic animals. However, no animal bite should be ignored; following thorough cleaning of the wound, any traveller should seek expert advice on the possibility of rabies in the area.

In Britain, the country's restrictive policy has been notably successful since 1902, when the last indigenous case of rabies was reported in Wales. Some 18 cases have been imported since then, including in 1986 a British lady living in Lusaka, Zambia, who was bitten on the arm and forearm when attempting to stop her own dog fighting with a stray. Not seeking medical attention because she wrongly thought she had been bitten by her own dog, which was immunised against rabies, she travelled to Britain and later died from the disease. Almost all other imported cases have followed dog bites in the Indian sub-continent, with one from Indonesia being the only exception.

7

Control and Protection

To understand the *spread* of communicable disease is the first step to achieving its *control*, which is why such detailed attention has been given to the subject in the last chapter. Perfect prevention of spread would mean perfect control of infectious disease. Then, once no-one is infected, there would be no infection to pass on. So far, unfortunately, the only disease to have been tackled with such complete success is smallpox, but the principles remain for the others.

To achieve control of an infectious disease, whether on a local or a global scale, it is necessary to:

- *eliminate reservoirs of infection*, by finding and treating infected humans, and isolating and quarantining them if necessary; and, if the reservoirs are in animals, make the decision whether it is necessary to destroy them;
- *block the pathway* through which the disease is transmitted, through personal and public hygiene and sanitary endeavours, and modify any environmental features which favour pathogenic

organisms and their vectors at the expense of man, the host; and to

- *protect and treat* those who are susceptible to the disease, using techniques of immunisation as well as chemical agents for the prevention and treatment of disease.

In this chapter a wide variety of control measures, grouped by mode of spread, are reviewed, and the next chapter considers immunisation and drug therapy.

CONTROL OF INTESTINAL INFECTIONS

Intestinal infections are prevented, and their spread controlled, by interrupting the chain of events that permits faecal matter and other pathogenic material to reach the mouth and be ingested. Faeces must be safely disposed of, human and animal reservoirs of gastrointestinal disease must be treated, clean water must be provided, and food must be protected from contamination by vectors such as flies and by unhygienic preparation and handling.

To achieve these objectives, great changes in the pattern of infectious disease have been brought about by pioneering reformers without scientific training, let alone a medical education (for what that was worth in earlier times). Many of the changes they wrought were in the face of entrenched opinion. Some, indeed, were based on a wholly incorrect appreciation of the natural history of the sicknesses they were trying to get to grips with. It was the essential pragmatism of these men which showed their contemporaries that the measures they were recommending – never mind that the underlying theories may have been fallacious – worked. And among the most crucially important measures that they forced into action were the provision for the mass of people of a supply of clean, pure water, and the implementation of arrangements for the sanitary disposal of community wastes.

It takes considerable effort, after all the years that have now passed, to conceive of the strength of character required by a senior and respected citizen who would risk his name and his reputation, and the scorn of his peers, in concentrating his life's work on such mundane matters as ensuring that faeces are flushed away – hardly the furnace in which Nobel Prize citations are forged.

In the developed world, the sanitary revolution fomented by these men is essentially over. Any of the diseases spread by the transmission of faeces to the mouth, and which require a substantial dose of the infecting organism in order that the infection may take hold, are now exceedingly unlikely to cause widespread illness. This is because water supplies, even in country areas, almost all come through piped supplies and are free from bacteria, and the treatment of sewage is aimed at minimising the pollution of sea shores, rivers, and other sources of water.

But just because man seems to have reached a generally satisfactory level of control in his efforts to limit the incidence of intestinal disorders does not mean that vigilance can be relaxed. Many existing sewerage systems have been in place for a very long time, and need a high degree of maintenance or even replacement, and this does not come cheaply. Floods after storms can overload the capacity of drainage systems to keep water separated from faecal matter, and in times of

other natural disaster or of war, or even through strikes, the efficiency of public services is inevitably put under threat. Contamination of some of the food we buy – and especially poultry meat by salmonellae – is now a fact of daily life, and many other aspects of food and personal hygiene in public places and in the home are poorly understood and commonly neglected.

All this, therefore, justifies the attention we now turn to the prevention and control of intestinal infection, and in doing so we take into account the special difficulties faced by the less rich and favoured areas and nations, because the problems they have to tackle are the problems we need to keep in mind lest our present controls weaken. Further, there is two-way traffic between these nations and the richer ones; migrants move to more promising localities for work, perhaps carrying disorders they picked up at home, and on their way they cross paths with travellers from prosperous regions who enjoy the thrill and adventure of visiting exotic places, meeting the people, and sharing their food and drink. It is as well that all should be aware of the presence or absence of control measures, because knowledge about the fundamental principles of disease control and food hygiene is often the only element the traveller can rely on for any protection outside the very cleanest and best-managed communities.

The disposal of sewage

Human excrement is an important source of pathogenic micro-organisms, including bacteria, viruses and protozoa, which cause not only transitory vomiting and diarrhoea ('acute gastro-enteritis') but also many more serious, long-lasting diseases.

Faeces are attractive to flies, which can complete part of their breeding cycle (the maggot stages) within them. The indiscriminate disposal of faeces is offensive to the senses of sight and smell, and threatens a community's self-esteem. Scattered or haphazard defaecation not only contaminates the ground where people walk and children play, it can cause pollution of crops and water supplies both directly and indirectly.

In most developing countries inadequately treated sewage creates effluents and solid wastes that are a threat to human health. When these wastes are spread on cultivated agricultural land, or used in irrigation systems, they pose a direct threat of infection, contaminate vegetables, and infect animals and intermediate hosts.

If the disposal of excreta is to be safe, then the following must be prevented:

- direct contact between faeces and man;

- the contamination of underground or surface waters which may be used for drinking or washing;

- access by animals or insects to faecal matter;

- any contact between excreta and food;

- the creation of a public or private nuisance.

If disposal is to be adequate, then every household must have access to a safe system for the disposal of excreta. In the developing world, methods for the disposal of sewage – excreta plus waste water – should be simple and inexpensive to make and to use in relation to the available resources of the community, and acceptable to prevailing cultural beliefs. As it happens, over the millennia the practices of some ethnic groups, and the religious observances of particular faiths, have developed with a view specifically to hygiene. Under some faiths, for example, it is customary to use different hands for personal cleansing and for the preparation and eating of food.

People may still have to learn to appreciate and use properly sewage disposal systems, even when provided. In parts of Mexico, for example, within yards of luxury tourist hotels, the local people are accustomed to defaecate on seaside rocks and beaches, and not often below the tide line. The ideal situation is that every family has its own facilities, and that they should be clean and maintained in good working order; but this ideal may be well short of realisation even in the developed world, in the poorer areas and worst slums.

Unless such facilities are well constructed and maintained, they can themselves be important sources of infection. There are particular problems with the selection and construction of sanitation systems for high-density, low-income urban areas, especially where squatters settle, and the prevalence of helminthic infections has been found to be higher in urban latrine-users in the developing world than among rural people with no latrines at all. Further, squatter areas often exist in places which are subject to flooding, thus putting further strain on an already strained system of sanitation.

In western cities the use of domestic water closets became widespread at around the turn of the century, and London's original installation of glazed earthenware sewers laid underground was widely copied. The next step was to limit the outfall of untreated sewage into the rivers and sea, and so treatment of the discharges in sewage farms was introduced, slowly to become almost universal throughout Europe. In some countries, however, untreated or partially treated sewage is still ducted into harbours or out to sea (and sometimes not very far, either), a far from satisfactory practice for countries which regard themselves as civilized.

The purpose of sewage treatment plants is to remove from the incoming watery flow the proportionately tiny part of it which consists of solid matter and contaminating micro-organisms, and so purify the water that it can be used over again. There are two main stages in this process: physical separation and screening of the waste water, and bacterial treatment of it. In the first stage, the coarsely-filtered water flows through a settling chamber which allows grit and sand to fall out. It then passes to sedimentation tanks where other solids can settle out in the form of sludge. The water is then referred to as 'effluent', and goes on to be treated by bacterial action. One method is to trickle it through large beds of crushed rock, where colonies of slime, algae and micro-organisms consume organic wastes as the water seeps past. Such techniques have been superseded by others including the activated sludge method, whereby the effluent flows to aerated tanks and is mixed with sludge, the organisms within which then digest the remaining organic sewage. The water from either of these processes flows on to secondary sedimentation tanks so that any remaining solids can settle out. The final effluent is then treated with a disinfecting chemical such as chlorine and released.

Where communities can afford it, a third stage is necessary to remove viruses, detergents and other dissolved impurities, with procedures including the use of alum or lime for sedimentation and coagulation, and activated charcoal filters to remove the dissolved organic matter. Other methods for absolute purification include processes known as electrodialysis and reverse

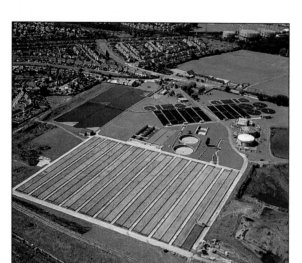

Figure 59 The safe disposal of faeces is the key to prevention of most intestinal infections.

osmosis, which can even convert salt water into fresh.

In the developing world, limited resources force the use of far lower technology methods for the disposal of sewage. They include buckets, boreholes, and water-assisted and chemical privies.

The use of buckets is highly undesirable, because it breaks all the guidelines for the safe handling of faeces: direct human contact is involved, flies and animals have access to the material, and the smells are offensive.

Other methods rely on the natural mechanism of decomposition of the faeces into harmless and inoffensive humus, during which process many human pathogens are destroyed. Complex organic compounds such as protein and urea are broken down into simpler and more stable forms, and the volume and mass of the material is reduced by the production of gases such as methane, carbon dioxide, ammonia and nitrogen, which are dissipated in the open air. Soluble contaminants soak away into the surrounding soil, and in a way which is analogous to that which operates in a sophisticated sewage plant, bacteria play a major part in the process of ultimate decomposition.

The bacterial mechanism may be anaerobic (shut off from oxygen), such as in the septic tanks which are used in many large cities even in industrialised nations, or at the bottom of deep pits. Or it may be aerobic, such as in the workings of compost.

Composting is a process by which under suitable environmental conditions aerobic micro-organisms break down organic matter to fairly stable humus, and it is of particular use in locations where even the presence of clean latrines does not solve the problem of infections borne by excreta because they are used to fertilize crops and add to the productivity of fish-breeding ponds. Composting encourages the use of all vegetable and human wastes as fertilizers while at the same time being a reliable way of killing off most pathogens. To be efficient, the process must be allowed to take three or four months, and frequent turning of the heap will ensure that it maintains the correct temperature of 50–60 degrees Celsius.

Disposal of refuse and solid wastes

Domestic refuse includes organic matter such as food scraps and garden materials, and inorganic matter such as bottles and tins. If disposed of badly, it smells, attracts flies which breed and can transmit disease, and provides an opportunity for the multiplication of other insects, mice and rats. The material it contains can pose the risk of accidental injury by cuts and puncture wounds, especially among children. At times of social strife, even in the developed world, measures to ensure the safe disposal of refuse can be disrupted. Further, anyone who believes that the disposal of private and public refuse is now inadequate only in the third world will find no difficulty in finding major cities in Europe which prove him very wrong. A visit, for example, to Palermo – for centuries at the very crossroads of European civilisation – will show how quickly neglect can lead to decay, while the refuse rots on the streets and pavements.

Refuse should be stored in securely-lidded containers of an adequate size, big enough to contain all the refuse generated between collections or removal. The surrounding surface should be hard and smooth, and thus easy to sweep up. Refuse should be collected regularly and systematically and disposed of thoroughly. Dumping in seas and rivers is common, but highly undesirable. Dumping on open ground, perhaps the commonest method in poorer communities, simply shifts the breeding ground for mosquitoes,

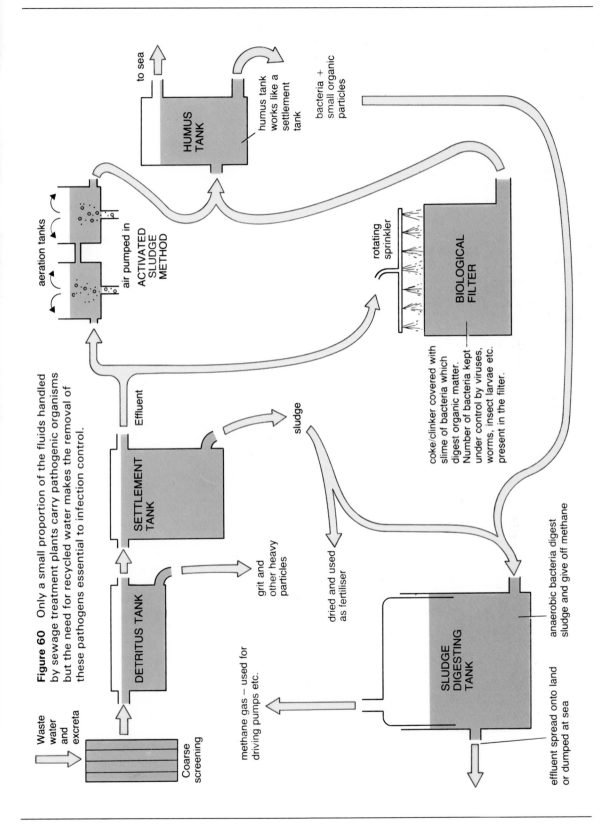

Figure 60 Only a small proportion of the fluids handled by sewage treatment plants carry pathogenic organisms but the need for recycled water makes the removal of these pathogens essential to infection control.

Waste water and excreta

Coarse screening

DETRITUS TANK

grit and other heavy particles

SETTLEMENT TANK

Effluent

sludge

methane gas – used for driving pumps etc.

dried and used as fertiliser

SLUDGE DIGESTING TANK

anaerobic bacteria digest sludge and give off methane

effluent spread onto land or dumped at sea

aeration tanks

air pumped in ACTIVATED SLUDGE METHOD

rotating sprinkler

BIOLOGICAL FILTER

coke/clinker covered with slime of bacteria which digest organic matter. Number of bacteria kept under control by viruses, worms, insect larvae etc. present in the filter.

bacteria + small organic particles

HUMUS TANK

to sea

humus tank works like a settlement tank

other insects and rats a little way outside the inhabited community. Burning, also common, hardly improves matters, unless it employs high-technology incineration. Composting can be entirely satisfactory under correct conditions with or without nightsoil, and controlled tipping, with spreading and compacting, is a method of disposal of proven efficiency.

The provision of pure water

Water is essential for life. It also carries the organisms which cause cholera, typhoid, hepatitis and the many others to which we have already drawn attention. It can provide a home for vectors essential to the survival of a wide variety of protozoal pathogens. On the other hand, shortage of water can encourage the diseases of dirt, including skin infections and trachoma.

Water is required for drinking and cooking, for washing the body and clothes, for cleaning up the immediate environment and flushing wastes, and for both domestic and large-scale agriculture. For such purposes an individual needs a minimum of 20 to 40 litres a day, with unrestricted usage in the order of 200 to 400 litres a day for each person being customary in urban areas of the developed world. Industry takes an enormous amount of water, with about a quarter of a million litres of water required for the manufacture of a single car. But clean water, like clean air, is not a limitless resource.

Sources of water include rain, ground water such as rivers, streams, ponds and the sea, and underground water from wells and springs. Rain is pure, but can be contaminated by the surfaces on which it is collected. Surface water is easily polluted by human and animal activity. Wells vary: shallow ones can be polluted by contaminants seeping from the surface, whereas deep ones are more easily protected.

It is highly desirable that water be carried into every home in pipes, an ideal far short of realisation even in many European countries, being practicable only in fairly dense settlements. Water in the home encourages bathing and the frequent washing of hands, and makes the washing of clothes a great deal easier. In the kitchen, fruit and vegetables can be freely washed and utensils used for the preparation of food adequately cleaned.

In rural tropical areas a long walk to the water supply encourages defaecation in the fields, possibly close to wells and bores.

The provision of pure water requires a substantial degree of social organisation, and the choice of an appropriate level of technology and its application has to be consistent with the socioeconomic and cultural attitudes of the people concerned. This has been one of the main considerations of the international charitable agencies during the 1980s, which were designated as the 'International Drinking Water Supply and Sanitation Decade'. Every community needs a safe and adequate supply of water (and would prefer an abundant one), but the methods used to achieve this must be affordable as well as technically sound, and in many parts of the world it is essential that all machinery be simple and easy to maintain. Even in the most highly civilized communities clean water is hard to guarantee, as old equipment deteriorates, and new obstacles are recognised, such as the ability of many viruses to survive purification systems.

Man's need for water puts continual pressure on our capacity to provide it, and the cleaning and re-use of water is constantly being extended. Two-thirds of London's water comes out of the Thames, and by the time it is taken for purification it has already been through the water treatment plants of several towns further up the Thames Valley.

Methods for the treatment of water continue to evolve over the years, but to achieve the basic requirements – freedom from colour and organisms, and clarity – the essential features are still filtration, sedimentation and disinfection with chlorine or other disinfectant. There is currently some interest in non-chlorine disinfectants because of worries about the carcinogenicity of trichloromethanes which can result from the reaction between chlorine and traces of organic material which remain in the water. However, an expert committee advising the UK Department of the Environment stated in August 1986 that they had found no sound reason to conclude that the products of chlorination in drinking water which has been chlorinated according to current practices increases the risk of cancer in humans. Therefore, the requirement that free chlorine be in the water is still generally considered highly desirable because of its proven effectiveness in combating water-borne disease, and chlorination is thus likely to remain the most appropriate form of disinfection in the foreseeable future.

Viruses, as we have commented, can survive

many sewage treatment processes including inadequate chlorination, although a sufficient level of free chlorine is highly effective in killing viruses if contact is for a sufficiently long period of time. Viruses are also inactivated by relatively high-technology processes such as heat treatment or irradiation, and storage in a reservoir for several weeks is effective if environmental and economic conditions permit it. Procedures known as flocculation can also be very effective, using lime or alum, but require careful supervision because the viruses may not be inactivated while they are being removed, and highly alkaline conditions must be maintained.

At the domestic level, boiling is a very efficient method of purifying even grossly contaminated water. Whatever the environmental conditions, water used for the feeding of infants should be boiled, and boiling can be useful when there is doubt on purity such as when travelling or during the breakdown of public facilities.

Food handling and preparation

Clean food, free of pathogens, is a necessary prerequisite for health. But in spite of legislative and technological countermeasures, the incidence of reported food-borne illnesses appears to be increasing even in developed nations. At every stage of production, storage, distribution, preparation, cooking and re-storage, the potential exists for the invasion of pathogens into food, and intensive modern methods for the mass production and distribution of food have provided yet more opportunities for infection. Ceaseless attention to detail is necessary, as the examples of food poisoning to which we have already referred bear witness. The appearance of food is no warning; most contaminated food looks, smells and tastes quite normal.

The prevention of food 'poisoning' is a matter of ensuring the highest possible standards of hygiene, from farm to abattoir and from market to kitchen. In the design of catering establishments especial attention must be paid to the disposal of waste material, so that its movement does not cross or interfere with the preparation of food. This problem is of great concern to any mass catering organisation including hospitals and old people's homes. Until 1987 hospitals were exempt, under Crown Immunity, from legislation designed to safeguard the public from the effects of unhygienic catering practices. The removal of this exemption was a direct result of the outbreak of food poisoning at Stanley Royd Hospital in 1984 in which 49 patients died. Intermittent outbreaks of food poisoning have occurred at hospitals since then.

At the abattoir, great care should be taken to prevent the contamination of carcases, and these must be inspected for evidence of infection and parasitic diseases which can be transmitted to man, such as tuberculosis, beef tapeworm and *Trichinella* (pork roundworm) larvae. The deep freezing of meat to minus 20 degrees Celsius for 10–14 days will destroy many parasites other than bacteria or viruses transmitted to man by eating undercooked meat. Meat must be stored in a cool or refrigerated place, away from flies, rats and other potential vectors of disease, until processed or sold.

In the kitchen, whether catering for a family or a regiment, there are several basic principles to be adhered to. For example:

- frozen meats and poultry must be completely thawed out before cooking, because otherwise the flesh in the depths of the meat may never attain the sort of temperature which kills pathogens;

- raw food – and especially meat – must be kept apart from cooked foods throughout the entire process of preparation, so that the raw food does not contaminate the cooked; and different work surfaces and utensils such as knives must be used for these two categories if possible;

- vegetables, which may be contaminated by soil, should be kept separate from other foods on work surfaces and in the fridge;

- if only one surface is available, it should not be a wooden one;

- work surfaces and utensils should be thoroughly cleaned on a daily basis;

- hot food should be maintained really hot, over about 65 degrees Celsius, and eaten within an hour or so;

- if it is going to be kept, cooked food should be rapidly cooled and refrigerated as soon as possible, say within an hour or two, so that bacteria do not have a chance

Figure 61 In developed countries we use vast quantities of clean water for a variety of purposes and its supply is taken for granted. The diagram below illustrates some of the ways that domestic water is used daily in the UK.

The situation is very different in third world countries where even the supply of drinking water is insufficient.

Average daily consumption in litres (*l*) per person:

W. Europe N. America	100 – 270*l*
Third world	4 – 40*l*

Source: Water, Sanitation, Health – For All? (1981)

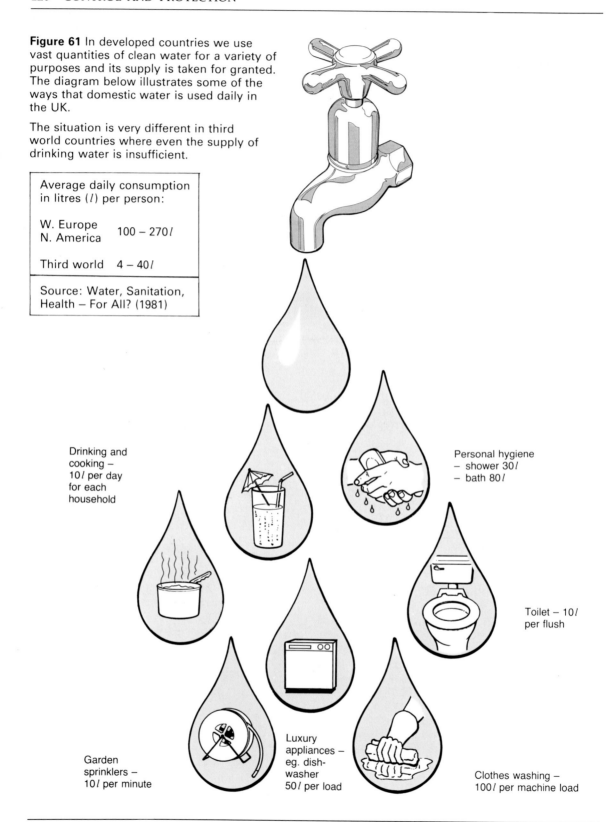

Drinking and cooking – 10*l* per day for each household

Personal hygiene – shower 30*l* – bath 80*l*

Toilet – 10*l* per flush

Garden sprinklers – 10*l* per minute

Luxury appliances – eg. dishwasher 50*l* per load

Clothes washing – 100*l* per machine load

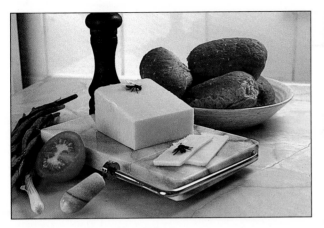

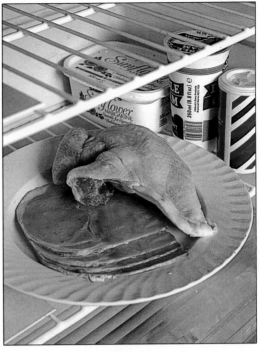

Figure 62 The principles of safe food preparation should be known to every person who at any time prepares or handles food, for example,

(a) Food should be kept covered to avoid insect and bacterial contamination and stored in a cool or refrigerated place.

(b) Frozen meats must be thawed fully before cooking and must be kept separate from cooked meats to avoid infection with organisms such as Salmonella.

to multiply in the warmth that so favours them;

- a large bulk of food should be separated into smaller units, to facilitate more rapid cooling and more thorough reheating;

- food being reheated should be brought to boiling temperature throughout.

The majority of bacteria grow best at between 15 and 50 degrees Celsius, but are destroyed at temperatures near the boiling point of water. Important exceptions are the organisms which form spores; these may survive boiling for several hours, but are destroyed at temperatures in the region of 115 degrees Celsius, for which a pressure cooker is necessary. Some organisms, such as *Clostridium perfringens* and *Bacillus cereus*, will form spores and survive the normal cooking process, but are not dangerous unless they are allowed to proliferate and produce toxins in food stored for a time in the warm.

Refrigeration does not kill bacteria. It slows down their natural rate of growth considerably, and deep freezing inhibits it almost entirely, but neither of these cold treatments has any permanent effect, and as soon as the organisms are returned to

a suitable temperature they start multiplying again. In commercial establishments a careful watch has to be kept on the actual temperature of the cold cabinets and freezers used for storage.

Further, a technique in which cooked food is rapidly chilled and thus preserved for later eating ('cook-chill') requires careful monitoring and the use of specially designed equipment if it is to be acceptably safe. A problem which can arise with the use of such procedures, which need painstaking training of staff, is that the people who employ them in practice (for example nurses) are not those who have received the training.

It is imperative that no food should be handled unless the hands have been thoroughly washed and dried, and the hands should be washed frequently throughout the preparation process.

Despite all precautions, the prevalence of salmonella bacteria remains a dilemma, and the preparation of poultry should be on the basis of an assumption that the carcases are thus contaminated, with the careful handling necessary which that implies. Raw, dirty or cracked eggs should be avoided.

When salmonella contamination of food animals is proved, it must be reported in Britain; as further control measures, protein feedstuffs should be sterilised, and all cows' milk products pasteurised. But in the case of poultry, it may be that the only way to ensure that the carcases are not infected at the point of sale is to irradiate them at the processing plant.

In the case of contamination by staphylococci, the toxin they produce is relatively stable at high temperatures and is not destroyed even by boiling, so it is important to prevent growth of the organisms and production of the toxin at any stage of the preparation of food. Man is the most likely source of the contamination, and a high standard of personal hygiene is necessary to prevent it. Fingers must not be allowed to travel from nose to food or from handkerchiefs and paper tissues to food. The mouth is a likely source of staphylococci; smoking should not be permitted in food preparation areas, and licking the fingers to pick up the paper to wrap the food is an unpleasant habit far too commonly seen.

All open skin lesions must be covered with waterproof dressings, and anyone with a 'cold' should not be preparing food. To prevent the formation of staphylococcal enterotoxin, food should be kept at or below 5 degrees Celsius, and storage in a warm kitchen at ambient temperature is dangerous because, as we described earlier, bacteria can multiply at astonishing speed under the right conditions.

Many viruses are destroyed by most cooking processes, but can contaminate precooked foods as a result of passage from a infected person's hands or droplets in the breath.

People who are suffering from intestinal infections must not as a matter of principle be involved in the handling, storage or production of food. However, meticulous attention to hygienic measures can reduce the risk of transmission of pathogens by infected food handlers to a very low one; the procedures used for the handling and preparation of food are in themselves more important than the fact of infection of a food handler. People who are not themselves infectious can transfer infection and contamination, whereas people who are infectious may not necessarily pass on their infection. Nevertheless, it is difficult to guarantee the necessary high standard of behaviour among all food handlers, whose everyday personal habits may vary widely.

In addition, some people who are involved peripherally in the handling of food, such as washers-up and managerial staff, will probably be using the same toilet facilities as food handlers, and if they are ill, especially with diarrhoea, they should therefore be excluded from food preparation areas. Food handlers returning from trips to tropical countries, or who have returned to work following a bout of infectious disease, may well require special investigation.

CONTROL OF AIRBORNE DISEASE

Diseases spread by the airborne route are controlled by isolating and eliminating human and animal reservoirs, ensuring good public hygiene and ventilation, avoiding overcrowding and the proximity of the infected to the susceptible, and by immunisation.

Most of these diseases affect the respiratory tract, which is just as exposed as the skin to pathogenic bacteria but without the solid barrier defences of the skin. Respiratory diseases are extremely common, generally short-lived and mild, and especially prevalent in temperate climates where people live, travel and work in close proximity. They are virtually impossible to prevent.

Droplet infection is, numerically, the most important route of all for the spread of disease in the developed world. When severe epidemics of respiratory disease break out, most communities will make energetic but generally useless efforts to block transmission pathways, from wearing masks to keeping children away from school. But to be truly effective, blocking the spread of respiratory diseases and other droplet infections would necessitate the complete disruption of community life. To take an entirely hypothetical example, suppose a new strain of influenza emerged which almost always had fatal consequences. Every individual and family group would be forced into a state of personal isolation. Conversation, travel, shopping, eating out: all would have to be proscribed. Being a disease caused by a virus, neither the use of drugs nor the wearing of masks would have anything more than a marginal effect on the rate of spread.

Fortunately, no such circumstances exist or are likely to. Such an extreme example is used only to demonstrate the impracticality of controlling the spread of these illnesses in the real community. Therefore, although in principle respiratory infections can be controlled by interrupting the pathway of transmission, in practice under present circumstances of urban life, minor respiratory illnesses are likely to become more common, not less.

Most respiratory infections go through a characteristic series of stages, and what chances there are for control vary from stage to stage. During the incubation period, between invasion of the host by the pathogens and the appearance of symptoms, an infectious respiratory disease is normally not communicable, although chickenpox and measles may be transmitted during the last few days of this phase. At the first appearance of symptoms, which for most of this group of illnesses are very much the same ('just a bit of a cold coming on'), the diseases become highly communicable. Yet at this time most people will quite reasonably continue to go about their business in the community, and thus spread the illness as widely as their travel and work habits allow. At the height of the sickness, if it is a serious infection, most people will stay at home or require treatment in a hospital, and thus only represent much of a threat to those who look after them. For minor illnesses, however, economic and social pressures may force continuance of a 'normal' way of life, meaning the continuance of community contacts. As the disease resolves, infectivity declines, but often not as fast as the individual's hopes of return to work or school are rising.

Some attention to personal hygiene will, of course, minimise the extent of spread. Droplets are expelled more forcibly and a good deal further by a hearty, unprotected sneeze, coughing, and a good shaking of the handkerchief before blowing the nose. Washing the hands frequently, and keeping them away from the face, will do something to reduce the risk of person-to-person spread.

Space, of course, is a type of barrier, and the more space there is between individuals the less opportunity there will be for airborne diseases to be passed between them. The converse follows inevitably: crowding makes spread easier and faster. In both world wars packed barracks increased the incidence of diseases spread by droplets, including some serious ones, such as meningitis. In the first world war it was shown that the prevalence of meningitis was directly related to the degree of crowding in huts used for sleeping, and when the proportion of men carrying meningococci in their throats exceeded 20%, then

cases of meningitis would start to appear. With improved and more spacious accommodation, the incidence dropped. In the second world war, attention turned from droplets to infected bedclothes and dust as carriers, and new techniques were introduced for settling dust and making beds without a great deal of energetic shaking.

Isolation was a method used in attempts to control the spread of this group of diseases far more in the past than now, except that it may be necessary still in the case of the most serious illnesses. The intention is to separate the infected person from other people during the course of the illness, and specifically during the period of communicability, in such a way that the agent of infection cannot spread directly or indirectly from patient to new susceptible host. It probably accomplishes little in the case of the diseases of childhood, which are now managed in rather a relaxed manner compared to days gone by, when periods of isolation and quarantine were strictly enforced. In hospitals, isolation is a special technique in itself, and this is discussed later under the control of hospital infections.

In practice, most infections spread by the droplet route can only be blocked by immunisation, a subject covered in depth in the next chapter. If the disease is caused by an agent with a single and stable type of antigen, and good immunity follows immunisation, then the chance of controlling the spread of the disease is good, and its elimination from a community is possible if the proportion who are immune reaches a certain level, a level which depends on the infectivity of the disease and on other social factors such as crowding.

CONTROL OF CONTACT DISEASE

Contact infections result either from direct contact through touching, kissing or sexual intercourse, or from indirect contact through the handling of infected matter such as handkerchiefs, bedding, clothing or wound dressings.

The chain of transmission is exceedingly difficult to block when social factors are as influential as they are in this group of conditions. In the case of the sexually transmitted diseases, after all, one of man's most basic instincts is involved. For other diseases spread by close proximity (short of sexual contact) such as infections of the skin and mucous membranes, and infestations by arthropods such as scabies, factors underlying the immediate causes will be associated with overcrowding, dirty surroundings and poor hygiene, in turn so often related to poverty and to economic circumstances which force a way of life only too happily changed if it were possible. Whereas a high standard of personal hygiene can in theory curb the occurrence of disease spread by close contact, in the real world the cycle of poverty, dirt and disease is a hard one to break, however good the intentions.

Although personal behaviour is an important factor in the spread of this group of illnesses, and in principle most of them could be limited by changing that behaviour, in actual practice to rely on behaviour change is an unpromising option for control. The prostitute who realises that AIDS can be fatal yet continues to work unprotected is saying, in effect, that he or she is willing to accept the risk of death in return for the money.

Hospital infections, the other conditions included in this category, pose especial difficulties in control because in any health care institution will be found children, old people, sick people and injured people, grouped in close proximity, and being tended by staff whose relationship with them is necessarily very close and includes the chance of contact with their body fluids and wastes.

If we are to get to grips with diseases spread by close and intimate contact, we are going to have to work very hard indeed.

Control of the sexually transmitted diseases

The transmission of a sexually transmitted disease almost always involves more than two people. One may transmit the disease to a second; but the first must have got the infection from a third. The more the number of partners, the greater the chance of infection. The risk of a man becoming infected as a result of one contact with a partner with gonorrhoea is in the order of 20–30%; in some major cities close to 100% of all prostitutes are infected. So, after five contacts, the chances are that he will have contracted the disease. Thus, the incidence of these diseases is highest among sexually active people who change partners frequently, and those away from home, including travellers and servicemen, are at particularly high risk.

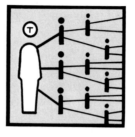

Elimination of human reservoirs

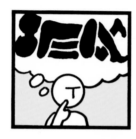

Discouragement of sexual promiscuity

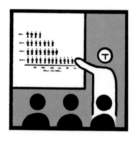

Education

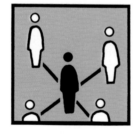

Contact tracing

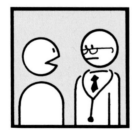

Early diagnosis and treatment

Figure 63   The control of sexually transmitted diseases depends on the elimination of human reservoirs, education, contact tracing and early medical attention.

In some communities a double standard of sexual behaviour encourages promiscuous behaviour among young men, including sexual intercourse with prostitutes, whereas the young women they will later marry are expected to remain chaste; and even after marriage, the same double standards may apply. Promiscuity before marriage, and infidelity within it, are both risk factors for sexually transmitted disease, and fidelity to one partner is a powerfully protective measure. Essentially the only reliable way of avoiding sexually transmitted disease is to keep faithful to one partner who is free from infection.

The general principles for community control of the sexually transmitted diseases include the following:

- the elimination of human reservoirs;
- the discouragement of sexual promiscuity;
- education on personal preventive measures;
- contact tracing;
- early diagnosis and treatment.

The reservoir is a human one, consisting of sexually active people who are infected. It follows that the identification and treatment of the most promiscuous individuals, including prostitutes, is the most important feature of this aspect of control. Screening and treatment can be offered to prostitutes, as well as to those who use brothels and bath houses of the sort where promiscuous sexual contacts are the most frequent. It is also possible to undertake a degree of screening among those people who are neither sick nor particularly seeking it: as part of the screening process for the AIDS virus in blood products, for example, or as is required in some countries the screening of serum for syphilis before marriage.

General health promotion and sex education measures can seek to discourage promiscuity by increasing awareness of the dangers of it, although this is not a measure with a track record of conspicuous success. In the case of AIDS, however, public education of unprecedented scale, cost and frankness has been employed in many developed countries, in view of the exceptional risk posed by spread of the disease.

Personal preventive measures are now encapsulated by the phrase 'safe sex' in the post-AIDS era, safe sex being taken to mean those sexual activities which prevent the exchange of the body fluids which carry the infecting microorganisms from person to person. These fluids include semen, blood, vaginal secretions, saliva and urine. The most important of the specific measures is the use of a condom throughout the sexual contact whenever there is a risk of transmission of disease; the HIV will not pass through a condom, and the device will also reduce the risk of acquiring syphilis, gonorrhoea and other infections. The risks to women are reduced by the use of a condom, and they should insist that their male partners wear one in appropriate circumstances. Further, a diaphragm used with spermicide offers a woman some additional protection, as also may careful toilet of the genital area with soap and water after sexual contact.

The provision of facilities for the early diagnosis and treatment of sexually transmitted disease is a necessary part of prevention, and they should be freely accessible and acceptable to all infected (or just worried) people. Such services should be confidential and available free of economic disincentive – free if necessary.

The tracing of contacts remains one of the most important associated procedures. Formal contact tracing is a system by which trained medical and paramedical staff interview patients and elicit names and addresses of sexual partners, and invite them to clinics for treatment. Less formally, counselling and health education can encourage patients to assume responsibility for tracing and referring their own sexual partners, but this process is of limited use if the patients cannot be relied on. Unravelling chains of contacts can be difficult among highly promiscuous groups, and in such cases the patient may prefer to name friends of both sexes who might benefit from interview and blood testing.

THE CONTROL OF HOSPITAL INFECTIONS

The control of hospital infections has become a subject for scientific study in itself, and whole journals and, indeed, textbooks are devoted to it. It is also a highly technical and specialised topic. Accordingly, only a few of the most important principles will be described in these pages; for those most closely concerned, there is a mass of detailed literature now available.

There exists in hospitals the potential for the spread of infection in two directions: from staff to patients, and from patients to staff. In addition, many patients become ill from infection by bacteria they have carried in with them as part of their own flora.

Every modern health care institution has its own procedures and policies for minimising the risk of infection, including the sterilisation and disinfection of apparatus, the disposal of infected dressings, bedding and other material, the use of aseptic techniques in the operating theatres and in the wards, the isolation of infected patients, antibiotic use, and staff education. In most such institutions widespread use is now made of disposable hardware, bandages and so on, in order to minimise the incidence of infections which were previously carried in reusable apparatus and dressings.

In many hospitals oversight of the prevention of infection is taken by a Control of Infection Committee, with day-to-day administration and control under the supervision of a Control of Infection Officer, who is usually a microbiologist and often chairman of the committee. This officer is likely to require the assistance of an Infection Control Nurse, who is in daily contact with the nursing and other staff on the wards. Membership of the committee will probably include clinicians of the various specialties dealt with at the particular hospital, representatives of sterile supply and disinfection units, and other senior personnel from the pharmacy, kitchen, cleaning department and so on. Agreed procedures should be in writing in the form of a manual, which will inevitably encompass an enormous range of activities because practically no aspect of the operation of the hospital will be free from the worry of preventable infection.

The control of hospital infection starts right back at the design stage, whether new units are being built or existing buildings and facilities modified and upgraded. Space, again, is a great barrier to the spread of contact infections, and the further the patients are from each other the better. Ventilation is a fundamental detail of design, and in some areas such as operating theatres and isolation units it is critical to infection-free procedure, because it may involve the deliberate arrangement of a one-way flow of air. Operating theatres must be designed so that procedures likely to release pathogens into the air can be separated from 'clean' procedures and, like the flow of air, the flow of people and materials should be generally from 'clean' towards 'dirty' areas. Kitchens, toilets, cleaning facilities in the wards and waste disposal systems should all be designed with a view to infection control.

Occasionally it will be the patient who is at risk from the nurse and from others, such as visitors and carers. This is especially true of patients with cancer who are receiving high doses of chemotherapy and/or radiotherapy. These treatments reduce the white cell count to such a low level that even the slightest infection could be fatal. Consequently extra special precautions require to be taken, including almost total isolation of the patient, until safe white cell counts are recorded.

Special care and, it follows, designated procedures will be required for some particular patients, and the procedures will fall into separate categories depending on whether the intention is to prevent infection spreading from the surroundings and staff towards the patient, or away from the patient to other patients and the attending staff.

For example, the Royal College of Nursing lays down published guidelines for infection control, both as a routine part of nursing care and specifically for the care of infective patients, the mentally handicapped, those in special units such as the emergency department and labour wards, and so on. If the patient is suffering from a serious infectious disease, and depending on the ease with which it may be transmitted, he or she may require a degree of special management varying from 'barrier nursing' with special precautions in dealing with blood and body fluids, to full isolation. Again, full and specific guidelines will be laid down by the relevant professional bodies.

In paediatric wards infection can spread quickly, and those children who are known to be infectious should be kept separate from the others. The newly born are particularly vulnerable, especially those in intensive care and requiring apparatus for life support, and very great care should be used in the drawing up and implementation of infection-control procedures. The same applies, in principle, to all intensive care facilities, and may include the limitation of use of certain antibiotics in order to prevent subsequent infection by resistant organisms. Patients being looked after in burns units will require a similar set of meticulously applied procedures for infection control.

As in the outside world, and bearing in mind that many sick and otherwise incapacitated people are now treated at home (so that principles similar to those outlined above must be adhered to), there are many simple procedures which can limit the spread of infection. For example, given that most of the organisms which will be doing the infecting have been carried on the hands, it follows that the chain can in many cases be broken by careful attention to washing, not only after using the toilet and before eating, but also before and after most procedures which involve touching the patient, excretions, fluids and/or associated equipment. The washing of the hands must be thorough, careful, and followed by equally thorough drying, as this is a major determinant of how many bacteria will be carried afterwards. Bacteria like it wet.

The use of disposable material for the management of incontinence, at home as much as in hospital, can minimise the risk of contamination of the skin of the patient and the attendants.

Masks will be used at appropriate times, with guidance in the infection control manuals, to prevent the shedding of organisms from the upper respiratory tract, and special clothing – sterile if necessary – may be worn.

Meticulous attention to detail is required for some procedures, of course, where to keep bacteria away is of critical importance. Every person, lay or medical, would now recognise this need in the case of operative surgery, but less dramatic procedures also pose a serious risk. The prime example is catheterisation of the urinary bladder. A few years ago, when the urine was allowed to drain through an indwelling catheter into an open container, the infection rate was virtually 100% after about five days; even now, with the most careful techniques, about one-quarter of these patients will be infected within the same time, and if continuous drainage is required for two or three weeks, most patients will eventually become infected. Catheterisation should be conducted with the same precautions as a minor surgical procedure, by trained staff using a technique by which they never actually touch the patient with their hands. In most cases the contaminating organism, when infection occurs, is from the patient's own faecal flora and transmitted from his perineum; if he is a long-term hospital patient, the infecting organism is likely to be resistant to many antibiotics. The most important single measure to reduce the chance of cross-infection by such organisms is scrupulous hygiene of the hands, including thorough washing and the use of a disinfectant, drying, the use of gloves, and painstaking aseptic technique.

Another procedure of high potential risk is the establishment of an intravenous infusion, which also should be regarded as a skilled procedure. Only essential drips should be set up, and, again, scrupulous handwashing and attention to aseptic techniques are required. Specific measures will be laid down by each hospital. In the background lie the extraordinarily complex measures which are now employed to make sure that the blood which is to be used for transfusion is not itself contaminated. In the developed world, these safeguards can now be taken for granted; but in the developing world, the transfusion of blood is a mechanism by which blood-borne diseases are widely spread.

The other way that infection can flow is from the patient to the attending staff, and a range of procedures must be specified in order to minimise the risk of that happening. Different staff run different risks, but over recent years the most detailed attention has been paid to two conditions in particular: tuberculosis and hepatitis B.

Hospital staff should be tuberculin tested (to show whether they have been infected with tuberculosis or not). If negative, they should have their chest X-rayed and be offered BCG immunisation. Only staff who are positive should attend patients with known tuberculosis or work with the tubercle bacillus in the laboratory.

The other great fear is of infection by the virus of hepatitis B, which used to be regarded as the scourge of dialysis and transplantation units, both of which deal with large quantities of blood, and in which several deaths occurred during the 1960s in Britain, the United States and other countries. Now, patients and staff should be excluded from renal dialysis units if they are carriers of the hepatitis B surface antigen (HBsAg). Laboratories were also potentially hazardous areas, but increasingly stringent precautions have lowered the number of staff who become infected from working with blood and blood products.

Patients who are suspected of having viral hepatitis should be isolated, and blood for examination treated with special precautions which will be specified in the appropriate manual.

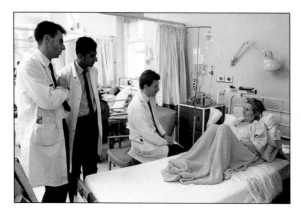

Figure 64   Hospitals provide the opportunity for the spread of infection between patients and staff. Every hospital will have its own policy for controlling infection by the use of aseptic techniques in the operating theatres and the wards.

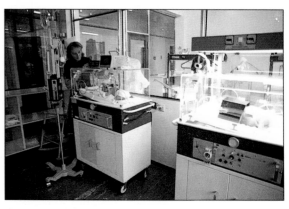

Figure 65   The newly born are particularly vulnerable, especially those in intensive care and requiring apparatus for life support, and very great care should be used in the drawing up and implementation of infection-control procedures.

Some patients will be considered 'at risk': drug addicts, known homosexuals, patients with tattoos, and patients from areas in the world with known high rates of HBsAg in the blood. Isolation will only normally be necessary if blood from the patient is to be handled or other parenteral procedures undertaken.

A recurrent problem is the use and disposal of what are known as 'sharps', including needles, intravenous transfusion sets, scalpel blades and glass ampoules, many of which will become contaminated with patients' blood and which can result in 'needlestick' injury. Carefully designed procedures for dealing with such implements should be introduced, and if staff are injured they should report immediately to the appropriate clinic so that they may be offered passive immunisation with hepatitis B immunoglobulin, and active immunisation as noted below. It is not possible to screen all patients, so the safest course is to avoid contamination of the skin with any blood or blood product, and wash any off as soon as possible. Operating theatre staff need to take special precautions if surgery is being undertaken on a patient who is a known or suspected carrier of HBsAg.

Human derived vaccine has been available for many years, but a vaccine for active immunisation against hepatitis B has recently been developed, and trials have demonstrated its value and safety. Recommendations on who should be immunised depend on the general level of prevalence of the carrier state. In areas of low prevalence, those for whom immunisation is recommended include health care personnel in frequent contact with blood or needles, particularly in institutions where there is a known high risk of hepatitis B, in dialysis centres and in other places using large quantities of blood or blood products; laboratory staff working with potentially infected material; and dentists and auxiliary dental personnel who have direct contact with patients.

Patients may also be offered immunisation if they are in institutions or being cared for in centres such as those referred to above, as may be spouses and other close contacts of people who are ill with hepatitis B or are carriers.

In areas of high prevalence military and aid personnel and all infants may also be offered immunisation.

THE CONTROL OF VECTOR-BORNE DISEASE

Diseases borne by vectors, as has been shown, have been for many years among the most important health problems in the world. Despite great progress in their control through the use of chemicals, they still represent a serious threat to most of the world's population. While it is usually poor socioeconomic circumstances which can take the greater weight of the blame for the continuance and spread of these diseases, in a curious twist of fate it is also the case that large projects aimed at economic improvement can so upset the environment that many diseases, such as malaria, schistosomiasis and onchocerciasis, have actually increased in some areas. As economic circumstances change, people tend to move towards urban centres, and the increased density of population can lead to an increase in the number of vectors such as rats.

To apply control measures to 'vectors', incidentally, is taken to apply in a broad sense to both vertebrate and invertebrate hosts and to animal reservoirs.

Controls can be aimed at three components of the disease transmission process:

- at the agent (the bacterium or other organism), through destruction of the animal reservoir or isolation of the infected patient;

- at the vectors, through limiting their numbers by mechanical, chemical or biological methods; and

- at the host, for whom immunisation or protection by drugs (chemoprophylaxis) may prevent the disease.

The measures to be selected depend on the natural history of the disease and of the particular vectors concerned in each case.

Of all measures, it is chemical destruction of the vectors which has the longest history, the insect-killing action of the natural product pyrethrum, which comes from the flowers of the chrysanthemum, having been discovered by the ancient Persians. An amazing demonstration of the success that could be gained from the use of chemicals was the elimination of typhus from Naples during the second world war. The city was occupied by Allied troops in 1943, but it had been badly bombed and social order had all but collapsed among the half million or so souls living in the ruins, caves, and temporary shelters. Conditions for the spread of lice, and thus the rickettsia of typhus, were ideal. The first case appeared in the city in July 1943, and there were hundreds within a few months. Army personnel were immunised, and tons of DDT powder and blowers were transported in. The whole population and their clothes were dusted. All body lice died within a few hours and, for the first time ever, a typhus epidemic was abruptly terminated. No ill effects on the human population became apparent.

The spectacular success of chemical control measures for a while overwhelmed emphasis on

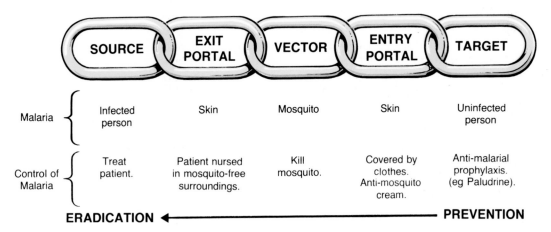

Figure 66 Control measures are aimed at the elements in the chain from source to target. The closer the control measures are to the source the more dramatic and effective they will be. As countries become better developed, they are able to aim their control measures further along this line towards eradication.

environmental management for the control of vectors and the animal reservoirs, and total eradication of many vector-borne diseases appeared for the first time to be possible. However, such optimism was premature. The chemicals had harmful consequences on other species which posed no threat to man, the vectors which were under attack became resistant to the effect of some of the chemicals, and public objections arose to their widespread use in the environment. Traces of chemicals which were found in the food chain raised fears of long-term toxicity to man and of upsets in the balance of nature, and when the cost of chemicals rose, they ceased to be quite such an attractive option from a cost-beneficial point of view.

Accordingly, vector control is settling down into a complex pattern of interlocking activities, extending from personal habits and activities to worldwide international initiatives.

The mosquito, inevitably, has been the object of the most energetic attempts at control, carrying as it does the causative organism of malaria as well as an array of arboviruses, together amounting to a ferocious assembly of serious disease. Malaria and yellow fever were severe obstacles to the building of the Panama Canal, but by intense attack on the breeding places of the mosquitoes, and by screening dwellings and isolating patients, both diseases were almost eradicated. The control of the malaria-carrying mosquito exemplified many features of the control of the spread of vector-borne disease in general.

The most basic antimalarial activity is fast diagnosis and correct treatment of the disease, and this can now be undertaken as part of primary health care. If people are not carrying the parasites in their blood, there will be nothing for the feeding mosquitoes to transmit. Country health workers can be helped by protocols which establish whether a fever is likely to be caused by malaria. Where resistance to the drugs by the parasites is becoming a problem, special malaria clinics are now being set up where blood can be examined under the microscope and an accurate diagnosis made on the spot.

Pregnant women are at special risk from malaria, which leads to a high risk of damage to the foetus, stillbirth, and death of the mother. In malarial areas, pregnant women are given a curative dose of antimalarial drugs when first seen, and a prophylactic dose thereafter. Infants and children also suffer badly, and in some areas children receive chloroquine as a routine. However, mass prophylaxis in children under the age of five years is no longer recommended because it may interfere with the development of natural immunity and accelerate the development of drug resistance. It is better to provide a system of primary care which identifies and treats the disease at an early stage.

Drugs are available both for the treatment of malaria and the prevention of the disease, and, again, can be administered at the primary care level. Chloroquine is the drug of choice for treatment, supported by amodiaquine. In areas where the parasites have become resistant to chloroquine, newly-developed drug combinations can be employed instead, and for some cases it is best still to use one of the most ancient effective drugs in the world, quinine. An antimalarial vaccine has been under development for many years and is in the early stages of testing in man.

While travellers and other high-risk people with no immunity to malaria are strongly urged to protect themselves from malaria with a suitable chemoprophylactic drug while in malarious areas, experience has now shown that only in exceptional cases has the large-scale prophylactic use of antimalarial drugs had a lasting effect on the prevalence of infection or the rate of transmission of the disease. Further, the development of drug resistance has been stimulated, and in any event it has been simply impractical to try to give the drugs to everyone. Where widescale chemoprophylaxis is being employed, such as in refugee camps, an energetic campaign of vector control should be undertaken in order to cut the rate of transmission and delay the establishment of drug resistance.

Control of the actual vectors is still, and will remain for some time, one of the main weapons for the control of malaria and, of course, the other mosquito-borne diseases. A flexible approach is necessary, blending personal endeavours, the use of chemical insecticides, and environmental and biological methods in a way which is best suited to the particular community.

To reduce contact between person and vector the net over the bed is still the mainstay, and it is more effective if impregnated with a longlasting insecticide. Doors and windows can also be screened, and burning coils and repellents can reduce the number of bites. A serious effort can be made to make dwellings proof against all kinds of vectors, with screens being supplemented by the plastering over and filling in of all cracks and holes against the ingress of rodents and triatomid bugs. The provision of footbridges over streams and canals in wet countries such as those in South-East Asia will reduce contact with parasites in the water. Safe, clean water and sewage disposal facilities will contribute in many ways to vector control, including the reduction of contact with snail-infested waters.

Insecticides can be sprayed on the walls of houses where people live, in order to leave a residual quantity of the chemical wherever mosquitoes may settle, or in outside air space in order to reduce vector populations quickly. Selective spraying of the lower parts of the walls of houses and cattle shelters is safer for the sprayers and more economical. A serious problem of resistance to insecticides is now developing, with the WHO recently reporting that some 150 species of mosquito and other arthropods are resistant to one or more insecticides. Indeed, many important anopheles species are resistant to several chemicals, including DDT. New ones are coming only very slowly out of the pipeline, as a result of stringent requirements for testing and use. Out of 2000 new compounds to be tested since 1960, only ten have been found to be suitable as residual insecticides, and the industry is becoming reluctant to pour more development costs into what may appear to be a high-risk, if not fruitless, endeavour. Another technical problem is the emergence of what the scientists refer to as 'refractory behaviour', whereby in a highly uncooperative manner the mosquitoes learn not to land and rest on surfaces which have been sprayed with insecticide. These and related problems are discussed at more length in Chapter 9, in the context of efforts directed towards the global eradication of malaria.

To an increasing extent the philosophy of using environmental management methods for the control of vectors, especially those which need water to breed, is becoming accepted again. Modification of the environment includes all types of drainage, which removes unwanted water from the surface; land filling, which eliminates the depressions in which mosquitoes, as well as the aquatic snails which carry schistosomiasis, can breed; and altering the topography so that, for example, water in hitherto sluggish streams is persuaded to run faster, which also discourages the blackflies of onchocerciasis. In particular cases it may be possible to manipulate the environment further, for example by regularly changing the water level of reservoirs, or sluicing out streams at times when the maximum number of vectors will be killed.

The developing field of biological control agents for the control of vectors such as mosquitoes and snails gives hope that chemical and environmental methods may thereby be supplemented, and the present reliance on insecticides reduced. All vectors have their own predators, competitors and pathogens in nature; the aim of biological control is to preserve these natural enemies and modify the environment in their favour. Sometimes, such changes can be very simple: for example, removing weeds from ponds makes it easier for fish to feed on mosquito larvae. More specifically, many pathogens and parasites are now being investigated, including bacteria, protozoa and fungi which kill mosquito larvae. In addition, several types of fish are being reared to eat larvae, and some also to eat snails. Neatly integrated developments make for enthusiastic community involvement. For example, in Indonesia, larva-eating fish are reared in trenches along the slanting edges of rice fields and themselves provide a source of food for the rice farmers.

Vector control of a different kind is exemplified by the control of rabies. In most of the world and especially in tropical countries the animal reservoir of rabies is the dog, and the magnitude of the problem of human rabies depends on the relationship of dogs to people. Effective vaccines provide a long duration of immunity, and it has been found that to immunise at least 80% of the dog population in an urban area leads to the disappearance of human rabies. Cats and cattle may also be immunised.

In the wild, carnivores appear to be the main transmitters of wildlife rabies. Since 1972 the WHO has been coordinating research on the immunisation of wildlife against rabies. Limited trials of the injection of wild foxes were not successful because an insufficiently high proportion of the population could be injected, but trials with oral vaccines have shown that these can be highly effective when ingested directly or on baits such as chicken heads. In Switzerland and Germany it has been shown possible to reach over 80% of the fox population in a treated area in a few days, and the advance of rabies has been halted in these places. An anti-rabies campaign started in Italy in 1984, based on the experience of Switzerland and West Germany, and appeared to have been successful in eradicating the disease in that country during 1987. Other European nations are now following suit.

Vampire bats kill hundreds of thousands of cattle in Latin America each year by inoculating them with rabies. It has been found that the cows can be inoculated with an anticoagulant which is lethal for the bats without harming the cattle. Another technique is to smear the backs of captured bats with anticoagulant and release them back into the wild, where they are groomed by other bats who ingest the poison. In pilot studies vampire-bat bites in affected herds have been greatly reduced, and rabies diminished or eliminated. Most other types of bat are not important carriers of rabies, and from an ecological point of view, one that applies to all aspects of vector control, it is important to avoid killing innocuous animals and upsetting nature's often precarious balance.

Figure 67 Selective surface spraying on the inside walls of dwelling places can be a safe and effective method of breaking the transmission chain for diseases borne by vectors, including mosquitos and bugs.

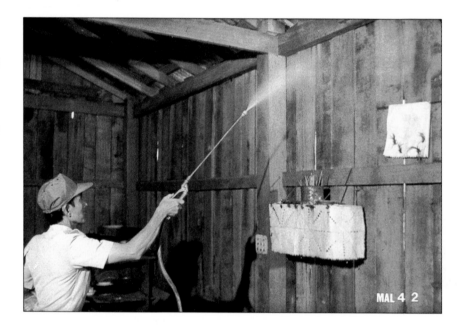

Special Controls

In the previous chapter a wide variety of approaches to the control of infectious disease has been described, grouped according to the way each is most commonly spread. There are some more general but equally important measures for the prevention and treatment of infectious diseases, and they are the subjects of this chapter. Immunisation, disinfection, sterilisation, and the use of drugs are all well recognised controls. Perhaps less well recognised is the fact that we can do a great deal as individuals to avoid catching and spreading infectious disease, and these matters are covered under the topics of travelling and personal hygiene.

IMMUNISATION

After Jenner had shown how smallpox could be prevented by the use of a cowpox vaccine, many investigators continued to study the subject of immunity in the hope of discovering vaccines which would prevent, or even treat, all the other infectious diseases. Although that particular hope has not been fulfilled, immunisation has decimated the incidence of some of the worst infectious

scourges known to mankind, and has been largely responsible for eradicating one of them altogether.

In Britain, the target level for immunisation against measles, whooping cough, diphtheria, tetanus, poliomyelitis and rubella is 90%. There has been a steady movement towards this goal during recent years, although the levels for whooping cough and measles are lower than for the others.

Also known (although much less commonly these days) as vaccination, after the smallpox vaccine named by Pasteur in honour of Jenner, immunisation is the process whereby the individual's immune response is either artificially stimulated *actively*, or it is supplemented *passively* with antibodies produced elsewhere.

Active Immunisation

Stimulation of the individual's immunity occurs as a result of deliberate ingestion or injection of antigenic agents. Just as if the individual had suffered an attack of the disease of which the agent was the usual cause, antibodies are formed in response, and the cellular immune response is also triggered.

An ideal vaccine, therefore, has antigenic properties which stimulate the body's full antibody response, but no pathogenic properties which would make the recipient ill. Like all medicines and all surgical procedures, vaccines carry some degree of risk, but no vaccine should present a risk which cannot be justified by the benefits to the individual and sometimes the community. Another desirable feature of a vaccine is that it be cheap.

The original pre-Jenner 'inoculation', or 'variolation', used pus from a smallpox lesion which, when scratched through the skin, gave rise to immunity by causing an attack of smallpox, but milder than a full-blown attack because the route of entry through the skin allowed less easy access to susceptible tissues than the normal route through the nose and mouth. But to make a safe vaccine, some way must be found to make the antigenic material non-infectious and harmless without at the same time destroying its ability to bring about the immune response. Also to be taken into account are the likely conditions of storage, including temperature, because long periods of transport in the heat may be necessary before vaccines reach their recipients. The smallpox vaccine was so successful partly because it could be manufactured in freeze-dried form, for simple reconstitution in the field later.

In practice, some vaccines are produced from inactivated (killed) organisms, some from live ones whose activity has been 'attenuated', and some from toxins which have been inactivated.

In the case of *poliomyelitis* two kinds of vaccine were originally developed, using on the one hand inactivated material from the virus, and on the other hand live material. The history of the development of the polio vaccines is closely associated with the names of the two men who took these different paths, Jonas Salk at the University of Pittsburgh and Albert Sabin at the University of Cincinnati, and with the controversy that surrounded the early trials. Salk had inactivated the polio virus with formalin, and preliminary testing in humans was in 1953 reported as being successful. Scientific thinking at that time was rather suspicious of vaccines made of live but attenuated material, with misgivings that living viruses could mutate to a more virulent form, and thus killed vaccine material was regarded as safer. With ironic tragedy, the first full-scale field trial of the Salk killed vaccine (which had to be injected) was followed by 214 cases of poliomyelitis, with 11

deaths; all the infections were traced to one particular faulty batch, which was withdrawn, but it took years for confidence in the Salk vaccine to be regained.

Meanwhile, intensive testing was taking place on a vaccine which could be taken by mouth, with the great advantages which that would offer for children and for use in the developing world. By 1954 Sabin and his team had prepared an oral vaccine using a living but attenuated virus, and it is this vaccine which is now used almost universally in Britain, preferably being given to whole families at a time.

In general, a living vaccine offers several advantages. The material producing the immune response increases in amount in the body and antigens are distributed in optimal amounts to the organs in the same way as if infection had occurred. This can cause some mild symptoms, but usually the side effects are less severe with live vaccines than inactivated ones. The immunity resulting from the administration of a live vaccine is one that can be relied on for many years.

However, live but attenuated vaccines can damage the developing foetus, and should not be given to women during pregnancy unless there is a high risk of exposure to a serious disease such as yellow fever. People whose natural immune responses are impaired, such as those with immunodeficiency diseases or who are receiving treatment which could impair the immune response, can suffer severe infection from a live vaccine and should never normally be given one.

Other live, attenuated vaccines are used to protect against yellow fever, measles, rubella, mumps and rabies.

The introduction of the *yellow fever* vaccine was the occasion of another rocky ride for a new protective agent. Several million American soldiers were immunised with the vaccine in 1942 before going to war; in an attempt to improve the keeping qualities of the unstable vaccine, it was placed in suspension with a small amount of normal human serum. Thousands of cases of jaundice occurred, with many deaths, and the yellow fever virus in the vaccine was blamed. As described in Chapter 6, careful studies showed that it was serum from a blood donor which had caused hepatitis, and now it is realised that the donor must have been a carrier of serum hepatitis, or hepatitis B. No such disasters have occurred again and, like the disease itself, immunisation with the yellow fever vaccine confers solid immunity, probably for life, although international regulations put a ten-year term on it.

The development of a *measles* vaccine was a major step forward in infectious disease control. The reason for immunising against measles, an unpleasant but not generally dangerous childhood illness which gives lifelong immunity and is worse in adults, is the small risk that the disease will lead to the serious complication of inflammation of the lining of the brain and subsequent brain damage. Even apparently uncomplicated measles can show changes in the electrical brain waves. The measles virus was first grown artificially in 1954, and in 1960 a group in Boston first tried an attenuated live vaccine in humans. Early problems with rather too active a response (the reaction was sometimes about as bad as the illness) were soon overcome, and it quickly became almost universally employed in the United States, with a resulting steep decline in the incidence of the disease and hopes of its complete eradication in that nation. It has been less enthusiastically embraced, however, in some other countries. It is not given to babies aged less than nine months or so, because the child will still have antibodies from the mother which would prevent the vaccine stimulating a full immune response, but it is usually offered in the second year of life. It produces active immunity in about 95% of children, with few unwanted reactions.

Because of the extremely infectious nature of measles, and the rapidity of its spread, epidemics are virtually impossible to contain. In order to prevent epidemics occurring in the first place, a very high proportion of the community has to be immunised, with studies indicating a necessary level of the order of 90%. This has been hard to attain wherever it has been tried, but if it could be achieved, then the spread would be greatly retarded, even if the disease was not completely eradicated. The immunisation rate in the UK was 63% in 1985 and 68% in 1986, with considerable variation between districts, a situation which is manifestly unsatisfactory. The introduction of a new vaccine combining protection against measles, mumps and rubella ('MMR') should help to increase the general level of immunisation.

Rubella vaccine is one of those which is given for the benefit of people other than the individual inoculated, in this case unborn babies, because the disease in itself is not a serious one. In Britain, schoolgirls are routinely offered the vaccine without prior testing for immunity, and in later life women are encouraged to have blood taken for screening for the presence of antibodies to the rubella virus. If no antibodies are demonstrated, and if pregnancy will be avoided during the next three months, immunisation may be offered at this stage. This entire process is an example of balancing benefits against risk: the whole risk, essentially, is to the foetus, and there is no intention to try to eliminate the disease by, say, immunising all boys as well. To do so would not be worth the small risk to them.

Immunisation against *mumps* is routine in the United States, where the number of mumps cases has declined by 97% since the licensing of the vaccine in 1967. In Britain there was once a feeling that the risks of widespread introduction of a 'new' live vaccine were insufficient to justify the prevention of such a mild disease, but the mumps vaccine is now incorporated into the new MMR combination vaccine.

Rabies is far from being a mild disease, and the introduction of a live vaccine for the prevention of infection of those who have been bitten has been of great benefit to people at some risk in endemic areas, such as veterinary surgeons in France and Germany.

All the above live vaccines have been viruses, but there is one example of a live, attenuated bacterial vaccine, the strain of the *tuberculosis* mycobacterium called Bacille Calmette-Guérin, or BCG. This is another vaccine with a controversial history, with a tragedy occurring in Lubeck, Germany in 1930 when several children died after having been given vaccine contaminated with a virulent strain of tuberculosis. As a routine in Britain, BCG immunisation is usually given at the age of 11–13 years after testing for pre-existing immunity, but children from areas with a high incidence of tuberculosis or who are otherwise at high risk may receive it at an earlier age.

In the United States other control measures have been deemed to be having a sufficient effect on the incidence of the disease, and effective chemotherapy is now available to sufferers. Further, the widespread use of BCG prevents the extent of natural immunity in the community, and thus the underlying prevalence of the disease, being assessed epidemiologically. Accordingly, in the States the policy regarding BCG has been different from that in Britain, with only people at particularly high risk being immunised.

We now turn to inactivated (killed) vaccines, which are used to prevent the viral diseases influenza, hepatitis B and (rarely in Britain, as just discussed) polio, as well as the bacterial illnesses whooping cough (pertussis), typhoid and cholera. Most killed vaccines are suspensions of killed organisms in some suitable antiseptic fluid. There can be no multiplication of the organisms within the body, and they cannot bring about a mild infection similar to the natural disease. More than one dose is usually required to assure adequate immunity, aided perhaps with 'booster' shots in later years.

In the earlier discussion of *influenza* attention was drawn to the remarkable capacity of the virus to change its antigenic nature over the years, and this has caused great difficulty in the preparation of a suitable vaccine. The WHO has set up a system of surveillance centres world wide in order to identify

Incidence of Whooping Cough 1948 – 1987

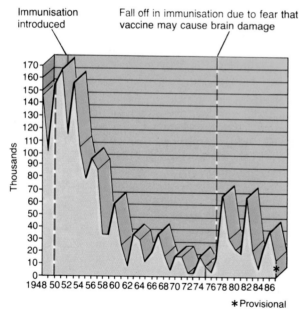

Immunisation introduced

Fall off in immunisation due to fear that vaccine may cause brain damage

Thousands

170 160 150 140 130 120 110 100 90 80 70 60 50 40 30 20 10 0

1948 50 52 54 56 58 60 62 64 66 68 70 72 74 76 78 80 82 84 86

∗Provisional

Figure 68 The proportion of a population which is immune to a disease has to be raised above a certain figure if the disease is to be brought under control. If the number of susceptible people increases, the disease can recur with renewed virulence.
(Source: Office of Populations Censuses and Surveys, and Statistical Review).

new strains as soon as possible, which it is hoped will be in time to produce a new vaccine containing the appropriate antigens before the new strain reaches the other side of the world. The chosen vaccine is usually offered in Britain in about September, in order to give protection during the winter months when infection is more likely and people are more vulnerable, but it is now mainly recommended for people with known chest or heart disease or who are elderly. Some individuals in key administrative or health care positions are also likely to be offered immunisation. Protection is quite good for the strain of the time, but it does not last until the next winter.

The *hepatitis B* vaccine is a new development, and its use has already been described in some detail when considering the risk of the disease to those dealing with infected blood and blood products. In Britain, it is now advisable to offer it to hospital and other health care staff at high risk of accidental infection.

Whooping cough, caused by the bacillus *Bordetella pertussis*, is a highly contagious disease which affects mostly infants and young children, although all ages can suffer. It has been recognised as a major childhood disease for centuries, and in very young infants causes serious complications such as pneumonia, otitis media, and convulsions with cyanosis and consequent brain damage. Although treatment with antibiotics is possible, the results are disappointing. Epidemics used to appear in waves, and were intensified by crowding and insanitary conditions.

Immunisation is the only practical way of preventing the disease and the deaths it causes, and mass immunisation is aimed at the protection not only of the individual child but also the community through raising the level of the 'herd immunity' to a level where spread becomes difficult. The vaccine is effective, as was demonstrated in Britain by Medical Research Council trials as long ago as 1959, and even those few children who develop the disease after immunisation do so in a much less severe form. In the United States, where a high level of immunisation has been achieved, the disease has almost been eradicated.

However, the vaccine is another of those which has at times been smothered in controversy, compounded by the fact that it is usually given at an age when other illnesses are common and may be blamed, by association, on the vaccine. It is certainly true that there is some risk of nerve damage following the procedure, but it is very small, being of the same order as the average risk of an adult dying as a result of taking a prescribed medicine. If every child in Britain completed the full course of three injections, about six cases of brain damage might be expected as a result, a tiny fraction of the brain damage and suffering which occurred each year as a result of the disease when it was common. During the mid-1970s there was a great deal of adverse publicity about the possible complications of the vaccine, including the possibility of permanent brain damage, and some pathetic pictures of brain-damaged children were shown on the television. The proportion of infants being immunised fell from about 75% to about 25%. The number of cases of whooping cough rose from a mere handful up to about 100,000 in 1977–79, with 36 deaths. Further, there was an associated fall in immunisations commonly associated with whooping cough, and as a probable consequence several cases of poliomyelitis occurred in Britain in the late 1970s.

There are, of course, children who should not receive the vaccine, including those with existing neurological and respiratory disorders, but the balance of risk for the population as a whole is clearly on the side of the beneficial effects of immunisation.

In order to establish herd immunity, which seems to occur as a very general rule when some 60% of the population is immune, public confidence in immunisation needs to be secured, along with frank discussion on what it can and cannot do. Each disease must be considered on its merits, taking into account its severity and the effectiveness of immunisation, and the dilemma

has to be faced whereby a course of action designed to protect the community carries a risk of harm to the individual.

Immunisation against *typhoid and paratyphoid* fevers has been available for many years, having first been introduced in 1897. The vaccine of killed typhoid bacilli can provide only incomplete protection, but the severity of any resulting disease will be reduced. Immunisation is not normally advised for people living and travelling in countries with adequately clean water supplies, but should be considered for those spending time in less favoured places. The typhoid vaccine used to be combined with vaccines against paratyphoid A and B as the combination called 'TAB', but the paratyphoid component offered little protection. Effective antibiotic treatment is available, and more effective oral vaccines are under development.

Cholera vaccines were until recently widely employed, but are now considered of limited use. Immunisation is of no practical value for the control of epidemics nor for the protection of people exposed to infection, but vaccines have been shown to provide some protection (50%) for a short time (three to six months) in highly endemic areas. It is not ordinarily recommended, and other measures can be taken in such areas to protect against infection.

Diphtheria was once the commonest fatal disease of childhood. It was described as long ago as the second century, but it was not until the nineteenth century that it became possible to separate one from another the various forms of childhood throat infection, many of which were described in writings of the time but most of which

Age	Immunisation
13 weeks	1st diphtheria, tetanus, pertussis, polio
19–21 weeks	2nd diphtheria, tetanus, pertussis, polio
36–40 weeks	3rd diphtheria, tetanus, pertussis, polio
12–18 months	Measles
4½ years	Booster diphtheria, tetanus, polio
Newborn (of Afro-Asian origin only)	BCG
10–13 years	Rubella (girls only)
13 years	BCG
13–15 years	Polio, tetanus

Figure 69 Recommended schedule for routine immunisations. (Source: DHSS).

were probably streptococcal infections, including the kind that led to scarlet fever. However, Pierre Bretonneau in France described the disease as a separate infectious entity in 1826 and gave it its name, and it was recognised as common in Britain and the new colonies of America and Australia. Following the work of Pasteur and Koch, the offending bacterium was isolated from the foul grey membrane which grows over the tonsils and the back of the throat in diphtheria, and it now has the name *Corynebacterium diphtheriae*. Soon after, it was shown that filtered material from a culture of the bacillus would produce the same lethal sickness in animals, showing that symptoms of the illness were due to a toxin emitted by the bacteria. A team at the Koch Institute including Emil von Behring, who won the first Nobel Prize for Medicine, started work on the identification of chemicals that would inactivate the toxin, work that reached fruition under the direction of Paul Ehrlich in 1897. After years of painstaking research he produced a stable, potent antitoxin and by the end of the century the mortality from diphtheria was already falling in a few parts of Europe and the United States where this was being used.

The development of active immunisation began in the mid 1920s, and was followed by a dramatic drop in the incidence of the disease. It is now very rare in the developed world, but it is important to maintain the rate at which children are now immunised.

It is only too easy to relax controls, when their very success has had the effect of reducing the public impact of a disease. But on a few occasions when diphtheria immunisation has in fact been relaxed, there have been rapid resurgences: in the second world war, for example, American soldiers in Europe were not immunised, nearly 6,000 got diphtheria and well over 100 died as a result.

The other form of active immunisation which has virtually wiped out a highly unpleasant disease is that which protects against *tetanus*, 'lockjaw', caused by *Clostridium tetani*, a bacterium which also releases into the tissues a potent toxin which attacks the nervous system. In most instances it has occurred when a wound has become contaminated by soil. Only a handful of cases now develop in Britain each year, and there would be none at all if all children were immunised and booster doses of toxoid given during later life.

The developed countries, including Britain, now lay down recommendations for a schedule of routine immunisations.

In the first year of life the triple vaccine is given, combining diphtheria and tetanus toxoids with the killed organisms of whooping cough. This is injected in three spaced doses, and is accompanied by oral doses of live polio vaccine.

During the second year of life the MMR (measles, mumps, rubella) combination vaccine is recommended, and at the time of entering school, booster doses of the toxoids and polio vaccine.

At 11–13 years BCG is offered to children who are not already immune, and girls are given rubella vaccine. On leaving school, polio and tetanus boosters are recommended.

In adult life, travellers may need further protection, and this is discussed in a later section.

Passive immunisation

Passive immunity arises from the presence in a person's blood of antibodies which have been produced by some other individual. If made by humans, the product containing the antibodies is known as 'human immunoglobulin'. If, as is now rare (because of the risk of serum sickness, a type of allergy), the antibodies have been made by another animal, the product is known as 'horse serum' or which ever animal name is appropriate. The protection given is virtually immediate, but it only lasts as long as the antibodies survive, which may only be for a week or two in the case of animal antisera, or a few months with human.

The most frequent use for what is commonly known as 'gamma-globulin' is the protection of travellers against hepatitis A, the form of jaundice which is spread by the faecal-oral route through poor hygiene and sanitation. People who live in areas where hepatitis A is prevalent are often immune, but people visiting these places can obtain about three to six months' protection from an injection obtained before travelling. Vaccines against hepatitis A are now under development.

DISINFECTION AND STERILISATION

When Joseph Lister was professor of surgery at Glasgow in the middle of the last century, among his adversaries was infection: infection of the bloodstream, infection of the skin and, most feared of all, deep infection of the tissues by the toughly resistant spores of the organism *Clostridium welchii*, which caused the foul-smelling, bubbling, gas gangrene. He had almost certainly read of the work of Semmelweiss, although he never referred to it in his writings, and he was deeply impressed by the observations of Pasteur on the spread of putrefaction by micro-organisms in the air. Cleanliness became his obsession; his aim was to keep the operating site clean in the first place, and further to prevent sepsis by using phenol (carbolic acid) in the dressings on the wounds and also, in the early days, sprayed into the air.

Towards the end of the century the principles he enunciated were refined by the work of Koch and others into a general concept of asepsis in surgery, whereby meticulous attention was paid to the cleanliness and disinfection of the surgical team, the patient and the surroundings, and to the sterilisation of the equipment to be used.

Pathogenic organisms can to a great extent be removed from the surfaces of people, including food handlers, housewives and hospital staff – and from their equipment – by simple washing with soap and water. The use of disinfectants does not eliminate the need for cleaning, and despite the message implied in some advertisements, disinfectants have no magical properties. Pouring disinfectant into a toilet bowl will not prevent little Jimmy spreading sonnei dysentery to his friends at nursery school; washing round the toilet seat with soap and water might, but it is not the sort of glamorous activity easy to depict on a television screen.

The aim of 'disinfection', which can be taken to include cleaning, is to remove and destroy some types of agents of infection outside the body, the implication being that the agents will not be exterminated but simply reduced below a number which threatens an infection taking hold. 'Sterilisation' implies a more absolute aim, that of killing all organisms or removing them altogether. In scientific terms this is impossible, and so for practical purposes a piece of equipment which is regarded as 'sterile' is assumed to be clean enough for the purpose for which it is intended, including procedures such as surgical operations.

Disinfection

The most important methods for disinfection are the use of cleaning, heat and chemicals.

Cleaning is widely employed and cheap. Organic matter is removed by scrubbing and washing with water, preferably hot, together with soap or other suitable detergent in order to dissolve oil and grease that may be trapping pathogens, and allow them to float free. Cleaning is often needed before other methods of disinfection or sterilisation are used, so that dirt and grease are dislodged and any remaining pathogens properly exposed to the disinfecting agents.

Bacteria, as we have already stressed, like it moist, and an important part of washing and cleaning, whether of hands or bedpans, is that they be really thoroughly dried afterwards, dry conditions in themselves being sufficient to kill many pathogens.

Heat will destroy all infective agents provided that the temperature is high enough. Boiling, meaning heating to 100 degrees Celsius for at least a minute, will kill most pathogens, and if maintained for 20 minutes will kill many spores, the armour built by many microbes to ride out adverse changes in their environment. An autoclave, which uses hot steam, can be used when higher temperatures are required.

Pasteurisation involves heat at a lower temperature than boiling and was, of course, first used for the treatment of milk. Special techniques, which include the careful monitoring of temperatures, are used in hospitals to disinfect items used in the wards such as bedpans. Other hospital equipment is often disinfected by steam at around 75 degrees Celsius in a chamber where the pressure is lower than atmospheric.

Chemical disinfectants are widely used in hospitals, institutions, public places and private dwellings, but their effectiveness is very limited if the surfaces to be disinfected have not been adequately cleaned beforehand. Some disinfectants act against some organisms, some against others, and a careful choice is necessary when it may be critical, as in the hospital or dentists' rooms. Also, the way the disinfectants are made up and used is important; the concentration must be correct, for example, and in some cases the temperature.

The main types of chemical disinfectant are as follows:

- alcohol at 70% concentration, used on the skin and flat surfaces;

- glutaraldehyde and formaldehyde, very active but toxic, used for disinfecting delicate equipment such as the endoscopes used for looking directly inside the body, including the intestinal tract;

- chlorhexidine, employed in the soapy scrub used by surgical staff before operations;

- the halogens, including chlorine, iodine, and hypochlorite, very active, used for cleaning up after spilt blood and for preparing patients' skin for surgery;

- phenol and phenolic compounds, of which a useful example is the hexachlorophane powder sometimes used to disinfect the umbilical stump of newborn babies in order to prevent staphylococcal infection; and

- the quaternary ammonium compounds, such as cetrimide, which has detergent properties.

Most hospitals and other health-care institutions will have their own established policies for the disinfectants to be used under various circumstances, and written procedures for the way the disinfectants should be employed.

Antiseptics are disinfectants which have been made up in such a way that they can be used on the skin, and they are sold as aids to the healing of minor wounds. They are, of course, no substitute for proper washing of such wounds with soap and fresh clean water. Several proprietary products used in the household will efficiently support the growth of pathogens while they sit in the bathroom cupboard, and it is highly unwise to assume that any 'antiseptic' products will kill all of the pathogens which may be infecting a fresh wound.

Sterilisation

Sterilisation methods include the use of heat, ethylene oxide gas, and radiation.

An example of *dry heat* is the incineration which is used to destroy soiled dressings and equipment which will not be used again. Tough apparatus such as some glassware can be sterilised in dry ovens.

Hot steam is an efficient sterilising agent, and the temperature will well exceed 100 degrees Celsius in an 'autoclave' under positive pressure, much the same conditions as in a domestic pressure cooker. Modern autoclaves are very efficient at exhausting dry air so that the items to be sterilised are surrounded only by steam, and are used to sterilise all equipment which can tolerate the heat, including clothes, instruments and some apparatus and parts of apparatus such as anaesthetic machines.

Ethylene oxide is a gas, very toxic, but a very efficient steriliser which will kill all pathogens

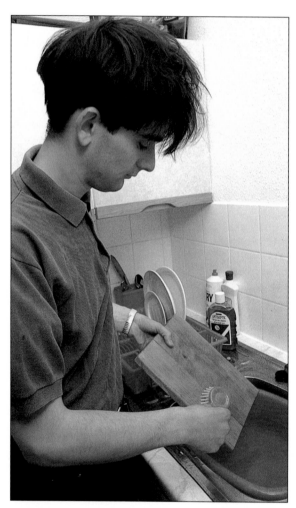

Figure 70 Cleaning and scrubbing are essential features of disinfection, even when supplemented by heat treatment and chemicals.

including those with spores. It is used to sterilise equipment which would be damaged by heat, including components from heart-lung machines, electronic aids for the heart, some respirators and so on. Some endoscopes are damaged by glutaraldehyde, and ethylene oxide may be used instead. Ethylene oxide sterilisers require expert handling, and are usually only used in special units.

Ionising radiation gamma rays, which are of exceedingly short wavelength but basically similar to light or to X-rays, are used to a great extent by manufacturers to sterilise equipment which is to be supplied to hospitals, such as needles and thread for sutures, catheters, gloves and so on. Radiation is an efficient killer of microbes, and may be used to combat contamination of food, such as salmonellae in poultry.

CHEMOTHERAPY

Chemicals now exist which can be used deliberately to kill bacteria, viruses, protozoa, fungi and metazoa; in other words, at least some examples from all the groups of micro-organisms which may be pathogenic for man. Most of them are given by mouth or injected; all have effects on the human body which are unwanted, but the aim is that these should be trivial in comparison with the desired toxic effect on the pathogen. The body's own defence mechanisms are usually necessary to assist their action.

The use of chemicals for treatment is called chemotherapy, and because of the specifically-desired action of this group, the medicines – 'drugs' – are known as antibiotics, or anti-microbials. It is now very hard to imagine medical practice without them being to hand.

Yet, with a small number of not very useful exceptions, they are a very recent entrant on the medical scene.

The development of antibiotics

Very few drugs with any activity against specific diseases were identified before the beginning of this century. In ancient times a number of rather toxic substances were used to rid the body of different kinds of worm, and Paracelsus used mercury to treat syphilis early in the sixteenth century. The first really useful medication was brought across

from the New World. The Peruvian Indians had long known that the bark from the cinchona tree was good for the treatment of intermittent fevers, and they demonstrated its virtues to the Jesuit priests of the new Spanish colonies. In powder form ('Jesuits' powder') it was used in Europe from about 1633, and in 1820 the French chemist J. Pelletier first isolated the active principle, quinine. In view of the immense influence of malaria on world mortality, quinine has probably saved more lives than any other drug, ever. It is still used for the emergency treatment of severe episodes.

There was little success in the chemical treatment of infectious disease from then until well into the nineteenth century, when at last the specific organisms which were causing the illnesses could be identified and brought into the laboratory. The booming chemical industry was able to produce compounds and variations of compounds virtually to order, and scientists settled down to find some that would kill microbes without harming their hosts.

Working with dyes, Paul Ehrlich found that some living tissues reacted differently to differing dyes, and in 1891 he showed that methylene blue killed malaria parasites. Two patients with malaria showed improvement after being injected with the dye. He found another dye which was active against leishmaniasis in animals, and then turned his attention to the arsenicals. First in rabbits, then in man, he discovered the effectiveness of arsphenamine (salvarsan) for the treatment of syphilis; introduced in 1909, with its derivatives it was used almost universally for syphilis until replaced by penicillin in 1943.

Following the first world war Germany lost its colonies and its source of quinine, and its large chemical companies set themselves to the task of discovering synthetic antimalarial drugs. Most of the immediate results of this research did aid the development of chemicals for the treatment of protozoal diseases, although not malaria in particular. One was called suramin, developed in 1916 for the treatment of trypanosomiasis; more than 60 years later it was to be the first drug shown to have any activity against the AIDS virus.

Meanwhile, prophylactic vaccines were being developed for protection against some of the great epidemic diseases, and much work was concentrated on the development of 'antisera' which could be used to treat active cases of disease. 'Serotherapy' had its few successes, notably in some forms of pneumonia and meningitis, but by 1940 all research was being diverted to different and very promising fields.

Even the most dramatic discoveries in science are preceded by years of plodding research, and a touch of serendipity does no harm. Such is the story of the antibiotics. Sulphanilamide, which was to revolutionise the chemotherapy of infectious disease three decades later, was first synthesised in Vienna as early as 1908 during some research which was following up Ehrlich's work with dyes. Scientists at the Rockefeller Institute in New York noted the Vienna findings and also synthesised sulphanilamide, and even reported in 1919 that it was highly effective in killing bacteria in the laboratory; but they never tried treating sick animals with it.

Meanwhile, in Germany, the whole dye industry was being organised into a huge conglomerate, and Professor Gerhard Domagk was appointed head of experimental pathology in the medical division of the group, IG Farbenindustrie. In 1932 Domagk hit gold: a substance called 'prontosil', which was a combination of sulphanilamide with a dyestuff, completely cured a group of mice injected with a lethal dose of streptococci, while all the control animals, which did not receive the drug, died. Soon after, similar success was being shown with human patients.

But outside scientific circles little was heard of prontosil, and Domagk's findings with the mice were not published until 1935. The reason was a wrangle about patent protection, with the German dye industry anxious to retain rights to the preparation. However, investigators at the Pasteur Institute in France, where there were no patent laws for medicines, had no scruples about making prontosil for themselves. They soon showed that the bacteria-killing part of the preparation was the sulphanilamide, which was free of patent, and so the rapidly expanding group of sulphonamide drugs was soon being used successfully to treat infections such as puerperal sepsis, gonorrhoea, osteomyelitis and meningitis.

The sulphonamides remained the mainstay of antibacterial therapy through until the early 1940s, and are still used today, most commonly in combination with another antibacterial called trimethoprim. Derivatives called sulphones are used for the treatment of leprosy, and other sulphonamide-based drugs are used for the prevention and treatment of malaria which is resistant to chloroquine. Even in the 1930s, however, enthusiasm was being moderated by the appearance of strains of bacteria which were resistant to the effects of the sulphonamides, and some of the side effects, such as disorders of the blood and kidneys, could be life-threatening.

Then a dazzling new prospect emerged, again as a result of serendipity reinforced by good science. Alexander Fleming, a reticent Scotsman, had studied the healing of war wounds in the first world war, and had become convinced that an ideal antiseptic would kill micro-organisms without harming the host tissues in the way that carbolic acid and hypochlorite solutions did. For years, then, in a small laboratory at St Mary's Hospital, he worked determinedly in pursuit of such a compound, concentrating in the first place on lysozyme.

Alert to any phenomenon which related to the destruction of bacteria, he noticed that while he was working with staphylococci one of a number of culture plates had become contaminated with a mould, Penicillium notatum, which appeared to kill the surrounding organisms. He grew the mould in broth, and showed that it destroyed several kinds of bacteria while not being toxic to animals. But his finding, published in a short paper in 1929, was seen to have little clinical significance, and the antibacterial extract from the mould, which he called 'penicillin', was very hard to produce in sufficient quantity for clinical research.

Meanwhile, across the Atlantic a Frenchman, René Dubos, was working with Dr Selman Waksman at Rutgers University, searching for bacteria found naturally in the soil that might be used to destroy pathogenic bacteria. He discovered chemicals which were highly effective in killing bacteria, and could be used on the skin, but which were too toxic to be taken internally by humans.

As the second world war exploded in Europe, Australian-born Professor Howard Florey was in Oxford turning his scientific brilliance and imaginative mind to the discovery of antibacterial drugs. He was familiar with the findings of both Fleming and Dubos, and his colleague Ernst Chain (a fugitive from Hitler's Germany) chose penicillin for further study. Chain managed to produce enough penicillin to duplicate Domagk's experiment with prontosil in mice, reporting in 1940 that penicillin was a chemotherapeutic agent, and the first trials in humans were reported the next year. Shortly afterwards, two groups in the United

States confirmed the effectiveness and lack of toxicity of penicillin.

But in Britain there were simply not sufficient funds forthcoming to develop ways to make penicillin in commercial quantities, and in 1941 Florey travelled to the United States to drum up support. Private pharmaceutical companies backed production with millions of their own dollars, and with the support of President Roosevelt penicillin joined the atomic bomb as the two projects with the highest priority for American federal government funding. Within two years penicillin was being used extensively in the British and American armies, and by the end of the war it was becoming available for general use as an inexpensive, highly effective and non-toxic antibiotic (a term which was coined by Waksman in 1945). Neither Fleming nor Florey ever took out a patent for penicillin, to the latter's reported regret in view of his chronic shortage of funds for research.

The reason for penicillin's lack of toxicity is its highly selective action on bacteria. The walls of bacterial cells are quite different from those of the cells in the human body; they are tough, and the bacteria cannot survive without them. Penicillin attacks the components of these cell walls while the bacteria are dividing, and because there are no similar components in the human body cells, no harm can be done simultaneously to them. But penicillin did prove to have two disadvantages: a small proportion of the population reacted in a severely allergic manner to it, and strains of staphylococci emerged which were resistant to its action.

The resistant strains of staphylococci were found to be producing an enzyme, penicillinase, which destroyed penicillin. These strains emerged rapidly in hospitals, surviving and successfully multiplying in an environment rich in penicillin and causing outbreaks of severe disease. The search for more antibacterials intensified, and new semi-synthetic penicillins were produced which not only avoided the action of penicillinase but also were active against a wider range of bacteria than the original drug. Also, unlike the original, some of the new derivatives could be taken by mouth.

Other groups of antibacterial drugs soon emerged, some from such unlikely sources as Fleming's mould. During the war the Rector of the University of Cagliari was searching Sardinian sewage for natural compounds which would have

an antibacterial effect, and discovered a fungus which did. However, he did not report his find until 1948, when it was picked up by Florey's team and formed the basis of a whole new group of antibiotics, the cephalosporins. Streptomycin, which was the first antibiotic to prove active against the tubercle bacillus, emerged from Waksman's study of micro-organisms in the soil; it had a meteoric rise to fame and success, but had toxic effects on the nerves of hearing and was superseded in the treatment of tuberculosis by isoniazid, which is related to a vitamin, nicotinic acid. From mulch in a field of stubble in Venezuela came chloramphenicol, and as its chemical structure was rapidly elucidated, it became the first antibiotic to be produced completely synthetically. Chloramphenicol was the first drug to be successful in the treatment of typhoid fever, and was also found to be active against the rickettsiae.

The tetracycline group were also developed at astonishing speed. An organism from a field in the campus of the University of Missouri was shown to have antibiotic effects in 1945; by 1948 the active principle, chlortetracycline ('aureomycin'), had been shown to be effective against an amazing range of pathogenic organisms, and at the end of that year it was marketed as the first 'broad-spectrum' antibiotic.

Antibiotics in practice

Antibiotics go about the business of destroying bacteria in several different ways. We have already described how penicillin and its derivatives disrupt the cell walls of the bacteria as they divide; the cephalosporins have the same effect, as do a few others. But antibiotics such as these can have no adverse influence on bacteria which do not have a cell wall to destroy.

Other antibiotics attack the metabolism of the bacteria. For example, to synthesise the nucleic acid which is essential to life, man uses folic acid, which he obtains as part of his normal diet. Many bacteria must manufacture their own folic acid, and sulphonamides block an essential step in this process of manufacture. Trimethoprim, used in a popular antibiotic in combination with sulphamethoxazole, acts by blocking another part of the process, so that the two drugs work together in a synergistic manner. Several other antibiotics work by interfering with the synthesis or replication of RNA and DNA in the bacterial cells.

Figure 71 Alexander Fleming, who discovered the use of penicillin to destroy bacteria.

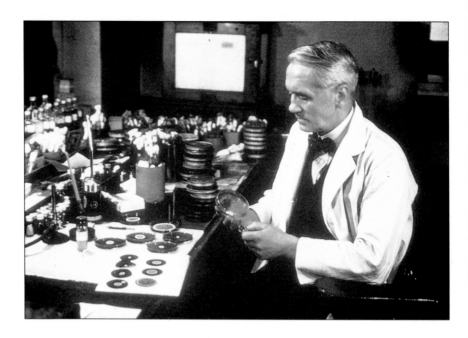

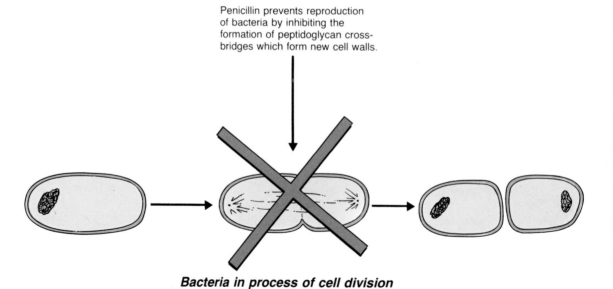

Penicillin prevents reproduction of bacteria by inhibiting the formation of peptidoglycan cross-bridges which form new cell walls.

Bacteria in process of cell division

Figure 72 Penicillin is effective because it destroys the walls of dividing bacteria, and it is safe for people to take because human cell walls are not susceptible to the same sort of attack.

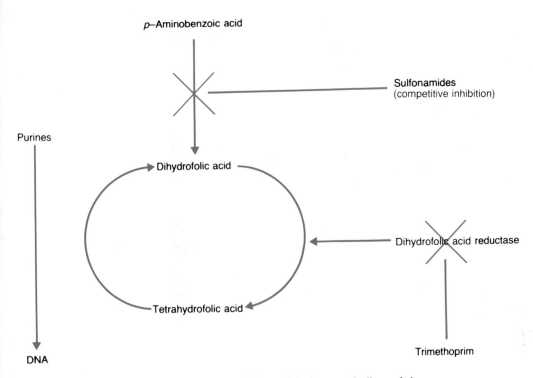

Figure 73   Some antibiotics work by interfering with the metabolism of the pathogenic organisms. Septrin is a combination of two antibiotics, Trimethoprin and Sulphamethoxazole which work together to block the synthesis of Folic acid. Folic acid is manufactured from p-Aminobenzoic acid (PABA). The Sulfonamide fraction of Septrin prevents this manufacture by competitive inhibition. It competes with the PABA to bind with the Dihydrofolic acid, thus leaving less Dihydrofolic acid available for use by the bacteria. To assist the conversion of Purines to DNA, Folic acid must be in the Tetrahydrofolic acid form. This is produced from the Dihydrofolic acid form by the enzyme Dihydrofolic acid reductase which is inactivated by the Trimethoprin fraction of Septrin.

The 'spectrum' of activity of an antibiotic gives some impression of the range of micro-organisms it might be expected to destroy.

Penicillin is a 'narrow-spectrum' antibiotic, with activity mainly against Gram-positive bacteria such as the streptococci; other narrow-spectrum antibiotics include cloxacillin and erythromycin, which are effective against the staphylococci, which are now almost always resistant to penicillin, and streptomycin and its family of aminoglycosides, which are effective against mainly Gram-negative bacilli such as *E. coli* and other 'coliforms', *Klebsiella* and *Pseudomonas*. Metronidazole is active against anaerobic bacteria and protozoa (such as those that cause vaginitis and pelvic inflammatory disease).

'Wide-spectrum' antibiotics include the tetracycline group, the penicillin derivatives ampicillin and amoxycillin, the cephalosporins, and trimethoprim-sulphamethoxazole. They are often employed when the organism causing the infection is not known, but this leads to consequential difficulties which are considered later.

Faced with an infection, the prescriber will take many factors into consideration before choosing an antibiotic. The first question will be, is an antibiotic appropriate at all? Infections with viruses will not respond, because viruses are not sensitive to the effect of antibiotics. Many minor gastrointestinal upsets are best not treated with antibiotics either, although there will be some sufferers, naturally, who are at threat from bacterial complications following these complaints, and antibiotic treatment is appropriate for them.

It is highly desirable to collect blood or other suitable specimens for culture and identification of the infecting organism before starting antibiotic treatment, because rational therapy is exceedingly difficult later if therapy has preceded the taking of specimens. When infections are serious, antimicrobial treatment can start as soon as the specimens have been taken, and early results from the laboratory can provide further guidance within a day.

The choice of an antibiotic will depend partly on the patient, with factors including any history of sensitivity to drugs, the possibility that the immune system may be compromised, the severity of the infection, whether any antibiotics have been taken recently, and whether the patient is pregnant or taking oral contraceptives (because some antibiotics can reduce the level of contraceptive in the blood and thus increase the risk of pregnancy). Ideally, a narrow-spectrum antibiotic should be chosen on the basis of the laboratory tests, because wide-spectrum antibiotics are much more likely to disturb the patient's normal distribution of bacterial flora and thus stimulate new infections ('superinfection' with organisms such as the fungus *Candida albicans*, flourishing in the absence of opposition), and also promote the emergence of new antibiotic-resistant strains of bacteria. In practice, however, some narrow-spectrum drugs are too toxic to use for mild infections, and broad-spectrum antibiotics may be used instead.

The choice of antibiotic will also depend on what is known as its 'pharmacodynamics', meaning the way it is absorbed, distributed round the body, metabolised and excreted. Some drugs find their way to particular organs, or work their way through accumulations of pus, much better than others, and an antibiotic will not work if it does not reach the site of infection in a sufficient concentration. Drugs that are not absorbed through the intestinal wall, for example, may be useful for intra-intestinal infections; drugs that are excreted through the gall bladder can be used for gall-bladder infections, and those that are excreted through the kidneys are useful for urinary-tract infections.

Resistance

Resistance to the effect of antibiotics, as we have already commented, is a major problem, and of course some bacteria show no response at all to some antibiotics. Resistance is one reason why antibiotic treatment may not be having the desired effect; others, of course, follow from the wrong choice or dose of drug.

There are many mechanisms of resistance. One, the production by some strains of staphylococci of an enzyme which can destroy penicillin, has already been described, and many other successful bacteria now produce drug-destroying enzymes. Some bacteria emerge with cell walls that are more resistant to being broken down by antibiotics, and some develop new metabolic processes which are not affected by the drugs.

In the laboratory it has been observed that some bacteria (without changing their essential nature) slowly 'adapt' to antibiotics, so that bigger and bigger doses are required to kill them. In the field, this appears to be happening with the gonococci, which were once exquisitely sensitive to penicillin but which now require huge doses to kill them. More fundamental changes can occur at the chromosomal level. The very fast pace of reproduction of bacteria can lead to the rapid emergence of mutants that are resistant to the drug being used, and these mutants can take over the infective process if they are allowed to build up to a sufficient number. When antibiotic treatment may need to continue for a long time, as in the case of tuberculosis, two drugs are used simultaneously, which greatly reduces the chance of a new mutant becoming dominant. By the same token, there is now a move towards shortening the period of antibiotic treatment wherever possible, which again gives mutants little chance to emerge.

Other changes have more far-reaching consequences. In Japan in 1959 the alarming finding was made that all at once strains of the dysentery bacillus emerged that were resistant to all the drugs commonly used at that time for the disease, and that *E. coli* isolated from the bowels of the same patients showed the same pattern of resistance. What was happening was that the genes responsible for resistance were carried in packets of DNA called plasmids, and these plasmids were being transferred from one strain of the bacteria to another. Plasmids 'coded' for antibiotic resistance are much more frequently found in places where antibiotics are employed indiscriminately, including countries such as Greece and Mexico where they can be bought over the counter at the chemist. Strains of *Salmonella typhi* can carry a plasmid coded for resistance to chloramphenicol, the only useful antibiotic for typhoid fever, and there have been several outbreaks of chloramphenicol-resistant typhoid in Mexico and the Far East. Newly antibiotic-resistant strains of bacteria can well spread from country to country, and thus the problem of resistance is an international one. Plasmids, and the changing nature of sensitivity within whole populations, are at least as important in influencing patterns of resistance as mutations by micro-organisms.

New antibiotics are continually being sought, and compound products can provide alternative treatment for a variety of infections, especially those caused by antibiotic-resistant bacteria. In hospitals polymicrobial infections and infections in immunocompromised patients can often now be successfully treated.

The general patterns of antibiotic use in the community, in hospitals, and in animal sickness and husbandry all influence the development and spread of resistance. With strenuous supervision and monitoring of antibiotic use, the resistance problem in hospitals is improving, although it will always be a threat and outbreaks of antibiotic-resistant infections still occur. Each hospital will have its own antibiotic policy, based on the pattern of resistance and cross-resistance which will have been observed within its walls.

In the wider community, such tight monitoring is less easy, and in some parts of the world impossible or regarded as unimportant. In principle it would be better that as far as possible infectious disease should be managed without the aid of antibiotics, because the more an antibiotic is used, the more likely it is that bacteria will become resistant to it. Conversely, when antibiotics have been withdrawn from use, it has been shown that sensitivity will return.

Further compounding the problem is the use of antibiotics for promoting the growth of animals, at which they are outstandingly successful, and it will be highly important in the long term that antibiotics used as feed additives for this purpose are not the same ones that are used for the treatment of human disease.

Chemotherapy of viral infections

The development of effective therapeutic agents for the treatment of diseases caused by viruses has been a slow business, in comparison with the early explosive growth in the number of effective antibiotics. It started with the discovery of interferon in 1957, which awakened hopes that virus replication might be inhibited. In 1962, idoxuridine became the first antiviral drug to be approved for general use by doctors, but because of its toxicity it can only be used on the surface of the skin or conjunctiva of the eye, where it is effective against the herpes virus. Soon after, amantadine was on the market, having been shown to be effective against the influenza A virus, with a prophylactic effect if it was started early enough.

Research in this field accelerated during the 1970s, concentrating on drugs useful for the treatment of diseases caused by the herpes viruses, with influenza and the rhinoviruses also getting their share of attention. Lately, the treatment of AIDS has become of critical importance, and consideration of the many other serious viral diseases we have described will show that there are several other important targets for antiviral agents.

Interferon was at first thought to be just one antiviral entity, but it is now known that there are at least 18 members of the interferon family. They induce an antiviral state in infected cells, they stimulate the host defence mechanisms and they inhibit the replication of most known viruses. They are clearly among the body's first line of defence against viral infection. In the early days of research it was difficult to obtain enough interferon, but recombinant DNA technology ('genetic engineering') has overcome that hurdle and clinical trials (controlled experimentation in humans) are now possible.

The common cold was one of the first infections for which interferon was tested. Several studies showed that interferon in nasal sprays had no benefit for treatment, but it did appear that it might have a prophylactic effect. Unfortunately, the most prominent side effects of interferon include nasal congestion and headache, so it could hardly be recommended as a preventive for the common cold! Several other and more severe side effects appear if the interferon is injected, and further work is being undertaken to derive less toxic interferons from the natural interferons or by synthesis.

Research efforts on antiviral agents have received the same sort of stimulus from the emergence of AIDS as antibiotics did from the declaration of the second world war. So far, however, the antivirals with the most promising effect on the AIDS virus (HIV) were all developed for other purposes. The first anti-HIV agent was suramin, developed in 1916 as an anti-parasitic drug, but it was found to be not very effective and much too toxic. Many others have been tried, including interferon, but success in the laboratory has not been translated into success in the clinic. Azathioprine, or 'Retrovir', which was originally developed for the treatment of cancer, is the antiviral most often now used in the treatment of AIDS. It inhibits the replication of viruses such as HIV, arrests the infection and improves the health of people with AIDS, but it does not provide a cure. However, it is very expensive and it is toxic, causing among other problems severe anaemia in many patients, and better drugs are urgently required.

The development of antiviral drugs, therefore, has hardly started. Rotaviruses cause gastroenteritis in countless children, the respiratory viruses are only too familiar to all, and the herpes viruses, HIV, and the highly pathogenic arboviruses cause an immense toll in mortality and morbidity. A WHO scientific group recently pointed also to the large number of other diseases for which there is some indication that viruses are involved, including diabetes, arthritis, multiple sclerosis, cancer and leukaemia, and the development of antiviral agents remains the major challenge to those who study the therapy of infectious disease.

Chemoprophylaxis

Whereas chemotherapy refers to the use of a chemical to cure a recognisable disease or to limit its further progress, chemoprophylaxis is the administration of chemicals (including antibiotics) to prevent the development of an infection or the progression of an infection to active infectious disease.

As soon as effective antimicrobial drugs became available, the use of them for chemoprophylaxis came under active research. Quinine had been used to prevent malaria for many years, and it was naturally hoped that the routine administration of antibiotics would prevent other forms of infectious disease. However, as would now be confidently predicted, strains of bacteria immediately emerged which were resistant to the antibiotic under trial,

which then became useless not only for prevention but also for treatment.

For mass prophylaxis, therefore, the only antimicrobials now used are for the prevention of malaria. Otherwise, antibiotics are used to prevent the emergence of infection among individuals at especial risk: the close contact of a child with meningococcal meningitis, for example, or the patient having a major operation, or the medical worker treating a highly infectious and seriously ill patient. Another group who take antibiotics as a preventive measure is comprised of those who have had rheumatic fever and have suffered damage to the heart valves; a further episode of streptococcal infection would cause further damage, and taking regular penicillin will prevent this.

INFECTION CONTROL FOR TRAVELLERS

The freespending tourist has been a godsend to the economies of many countries in the world, and the booming tourist industry is now a vitally important generator of foreign capital in some of the very poorest nations. Further, the growth of the package tour business has opened international travel to thousands of those who have never set foot 'abroad' before. What were once quiet little Mediterranean resorts now hum all summer with the sounds of people out and about, enjoying themselves, and package tour groups are now to be found in parts of the developing world that only a short time ago were visited only by the most intrepid and individualist travellers.

It will be apparent to even the casual reader of this book that most of today's more troublesome infections are to be found outside the countries of northern Europe, the North American continent north of Mexico, and Australasia, all of which share a high standard of living and a roughly similar general level of private and public hygiene. The tourist may well assume that the proprietor of a smart restaurant in Acapulco, Marbella, Mykonos, or Bangkok, together with all his staff, share his ideas of hygiene in food preparation and storage; but he could well be wrong. And the organisms which he ingests with his food and water will be strange to him and his immune system. Further off the beaten track, the traveller anxious to see parts of the world unaccompanied by

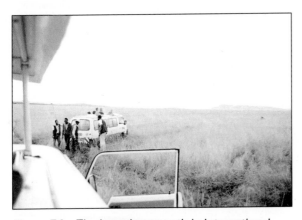

Figure 74 The booming growth in international travel has increased the likelihood of infection. An unpredictable environment is especially a problem for the overland traveller who plans his own journey. Such travellers need greater knowledge of disease prevention and its management than the traveller on a package holiday whose environment, food, and drink are largely in the hands of the operator.

thousands of others, and to share for a while the lifestyle of the people living there, will be exposed to the risk of infectious diseases which are virtually unknown in the country from which he came.

If he does fall ill while overseas, the traveller may have difficulty finding a doctor who understands his language, or medical care of a standard that he expects back home, or medical care he can afford, or any medical care at all.

Returning, sometimes within the incubation period of a disease he may have acquired overseas, the traveller may not recognise the symptoms of the illness he suffers once back home as those of an infection acquired on holiday; malaria, for example, can seem awfully like influenza.

To be in a position to take reasonable

Figure 75 The risk presented by different infectious diseases varies widely throughout the world, but the reporting of infections is of dubious reliability in the locations where they are likely to be most prevalent. This map indicates some particular problem areas.

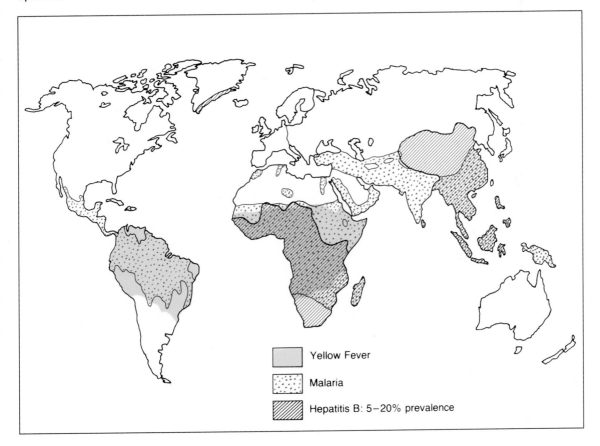

Yellow Fever

Malaria

Hepatitis B: 5–20% prevalence

precautions against infectious disease while travelling, it is necessary to know something about the risk of particular diseases in the areas to be visited, and about the way these diseases are spread. As is made clear throughout this book, it is understanding the spread of a disease which is the key to preventing it. The distribution of some of the commonest and most important infectious diseases has been mentioned at appropriate occasions in these pages, but a planned trip to, say, Guinea-Bissau would need the support of more detailed, up-to-date and expert advice, for which there are several sources.

The WHO publishes an annual booklet on international requirements for immunisation which, although aimed primarily at national health administrations, also contains advice for international travel. It gives detailed recommendations for the prophylaxis of malaria, with maps showing the main areas where malaria transmission occurs and where the organism causing falciparum malaria is resistant to chloroquine.

In Britain, the Department of Health and Social Security publishes a yearly leaflet with very concise advice on the reduction of health risks abroad, as well as another leaflet on medical costs abroad. Similar agencies exist in the other developed countries. A British Medical Journal publication aimed at doctors, *ABC of Healthy Travel*, includes a comprehensive list of sources of advice.

In London, an organisation called Medical Advisory Services for Travellers Abroad (MASTA) is based at the London School of Hygiene and Tropical Medicine and maintains a computerised bank of information on 84 diseases in 230 areas of the world. From these data it can prepare written advice for individual travellers, tailored to the particular health needs of the journey or longer stay abroad.

'Official' statistics on the prevalence of disease in the developing world are notoriously unreliable, especially in the case of the countries for which the information might be particularly useful. Further, the situation in individual countries, especially in relation to infectious disease, can change in a very short space of time. Given these reservations, the WHO describes the geographical distribution of potential health hazards to travellers in its booklet, and there is another compendium of advice from several sources, including expert estimates (as

opposed to official figures) of the prevalence of even the most obscure diseases, in *Travellers' Health*, edited by Richard Dawood.

Diseases spread by food and drink via the oral route, commonly causing intestinal upsets characterised as 'travellers' diarrhoea', are the most likely to cause problems. These can include cholera, the bacillary dysenteries, amoebic dysentery and giardiasis. They may also include infection by various forms of helminth, the virus of hepatitis A and other types of hepatitis, the typhoid and paratyphoid fevers, and salmonellosis. A 1977 British survey showed that nearly half of all international travellers had suffered some sort of illness while abroad or soon after returning home, and 80% of these illnesses were gastrointestinal in nature. Very deficient in the antibodies to the antigens they are bound to encounter, holiday makers are extremely susceptible to the sort of intestinal infections which cause neither the locals, nor more seasoned travellers, any real concern.

Travellers to Central America, the Far East, and the Mediterranean basin all seem to be at particular risk. In a nice piece of defensive propaganda, Mexico has labelled travellers' diarrhoea 'turista', thus neatly shifting the responsibility back to the traveller, who is then inclined to blame, perhaps, a 'change in the water'. The traveller would be well advised to remember that it is not the H_2O which changes, it is the pathogenic organisms which contaminate it and the food it accompanies, and that these organisms are usually lying in a small nest of someone else's faeces.

There are three intestinal infections for which immunisation is available: hepatitis A, cholera and typhoid, and all might be considered for regions where the traveller could be at risk, depending on his travel plans and the time he intends to stay in the country. Polio is also spread orally, and a booster dose may be a wise precaution. There is an obvious difference in risk between staying with a group in a resort hotel and trekking through the jungle.

The risk of all infections spread orally can be minimised by strict adherence to a few simple rules, all of which flow from the principles of control described earlier in these pages. Cooking destroys nearly all pathogens, and hot, recently-cooked food is practically always safe, even if purchased from a roadside vendor. Recooked foods and local attempts at 'gourmet' cooking are much less reliable, and cooked food which has been held at ambient temperature for some time constitutes one of the commonest causes of food-borne illness. Cold foods, especially those attractively displayed in the open, are highly likely to be contaminated. To be safe, fish and shellfish should not be eaten raw, which will disappoint oyster lovers and travellers in Central America and Japan. Salads and uncooked vegetables can be assumed to be contaminated with soil and whatever has been used to fertilise it, and the same applies to fresh fruits. These, however, often have a skin which can be freshly peeled, and are safe if prepared this way by the traveller.

Water is safe in northern Europe, North America and Australasia, and should be regarded as probably unsafe anywhere else. If the local ladies buy water in bottles at the supermarket, it could be a clue to the safety of the water in the nearby hotel. Bottled carbonated water is safer than the non-carbonated variety. Boiling renders even murky water safe, and sterilising tablets can be used where boiling is impossible.

At certain seasons, some fish and shellfish contain poisonous biotoxins even when well cooked, and the symptoms can cause vague and puzzling illness for many months afterwards. Fish in tropical waters such as the Caribbean are especially suspect, and it may be hard to tell when buying fish or eating out whether it has been imported or caught locally.

Infections requiring a vector for transmission are usually passed to the traveller by the bite of a mosquito or sandfly, except that the more intrepid will also face the risk of contact with infected snails and other vectors, especially in fresh water. The effects of mosquito bites can range from itchy discomfort, through the highly unpleasant sores of leishmaniasis, to the potentially lethal malaria, and it is much better not to get bitten.

In areas where bites are a problem, and especially where malaria is prevalent, long-sleeved clothes and trousers should be worn from the time the sun approaches the horizon. The use of an insect repellent such as diethyl toluamide ('deet') can be very effective, especially if aided in bad areas by wristlets and anklets soaked in a solution of the chemical. Sleeping should preferably be indoors, in screened quarters; if not, then under a mosquito net is best.

Up-to-date advice on the prevalence of malaria is essential before travelling into the warmer parts of the world, because preventive drugs will almost certainly be required, and the choice of the best ones for the particular area will depend on local patterns of resistance of the parasites to the drugs. The other arthropod-borne disease for which good protection is available is yellow fever, with effective immunisation mandatory by international health regulation for several countries of Africa and Latin America.

Diseases spread by contact are unlikely to be more of a problem to the traveller than at home, unless he or she becomes exposed to some extra risk of sexually transmitted disease. It is often stated that the relaxed ambience of travel leads to unusually uninhibited behaviour while on holiday, but the traveller should bear in mind the very high rate of sexually transmitted disease among prostitutes in many countries, especially in the Far East, and that many of these infections are now exceedingly resistant to antibiotic treatment. Diseases to which the sexually uninhibited traveller is now exposed include hepatitis B and AIDS as well as the more familiar infections, and to take a companion is much safer than to engage in casual sex while away. If the risk is taken, it should be minimised by the use of condoms and following the rules of 'safe sex', specifically avoiding sexual practices which involve the exchange of body fluids.

On return from a trip to foreign parts, a medical check-up may be of value, especially if travel has been to remote, hot regions, and if living conditions and food have been shared with the local people. It is, of course, not only important that the doctor doing the check-up be told of the regions visited or lived in, but also that any other doctor be informed about recent travel in the event of illness arising after return.

It is understandable that travel agents and others in the tourist industry are reluctant to discourage potential travellers by frightening them with the risk of obscure diseases, and that the advice they give is usually limited to regulations which must be obeyed. But the travel of a great many people would be a great deal happier if they knew some of these risks, and of the simple measures that can be taken to minimise them.

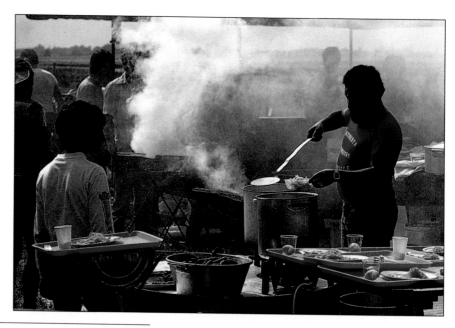

Figure 76 When travelling abroad, hot, freshly cooked food is likely to be safe to eat anywhere, as are fruits you have peeled yourself.

PERSONAL HYGIENE

In this book we have harped from time to time on the fact that a great many infections would have their route of transmission cut if a higher level of hygiene could be attained. Good public hygiene cuts the risk of the great epidemic diseases, institutional hygiene cuts the risk of infections in restaurants and hospitals, and good personal – that is to say, individual – hygiene can cut the risk of an individual contracting infectious disease and passing on a disease if he is carrying it himself.

Bacteria live and thrive in dead organic material. The surface layers of the skin are composed of the dead cells which are constantly being shed by the lower layers, and bacteria abound over the entire skin surface. They favour folds in the skin and the darker, moister areas such as under the arms, between the toes and in the folds of the hands. Especially common are the staphylococci, not usually causing us any harm, but making their presence known by the way that breaks in the skin surface are easily colonised by pathogenic varieties which cause minor infections such as pimples and boils. The same bacteria, or their close relations, can cause fatal infectious disease in those who are particularly vulnerable, such as newborn babies, those with deficiencies in their immune system, and the old and sick.

The mucous membranes are but an extension of the skin, and bacteria thrive in the dark, moist conditions found in the mouth, nose and throat, nourished by the constant supply of dead cells shed from the membranous layers. A new supply of microbes is constantly being added from the air, and from food and water. Again, as we explained early in this book, most of these bacteria – staphylococci, streptococci, pneumococci and meningococci predominating – cause us no harm, but they and their relatives can all cause illness if conditions are right for them.

The other part of the body where conditions are just right for micro-organisms to thrive is the bowel, where a large part of the bulk of the faeces is composed of dead cells and bacteria of the kind that live in the absence of oxygen. Again, they cause little or no disease when conditions are normal and people are fit – but the same organisms can cause devastating illness among, say, malnourished children, and they may be aided by truly pathogenic bacteria, perhaps sheltered in cysts and spores, which have been causing their current host no harm but which can cause severe illness to a new host.

As a simple matter of social conscience, therefore, apart from the pragmatic aim of avoiding unnecessary infection, it only makes sense to practise a system of personal hygiene which promotes health and limits the spread of infectious disease.

Diseases spread by the oral route would have their transmission almost totally blocked if faecal matter was not being carried on the hands. This might seem to be a fact which is blindingly obvious, but to observe the number of people marching out of public toilets without washing their hands is to observe that for many people, knowledge is not necessarily converted into action. The hands should always be washed with soap and water immediately after evacuation of the bowels or bladder. Soap has a detergent action which dissolves the oils and greases within which the bacteria may be lying, and which may well be resistant to an unaided flow of water.

It is important, too, to wash the hands thoroughly after handling material which may be contaminated with faecal matter, such as babies' nappies, a point which if emphasised during antenatal instruction could reduce the risk of unnecessary infection of the children. Bacteria and protozoa can survive on many surfaces for a while at least, and articles that have been used for toilet purposes by others should be kept away from the face, genitalia and wounds. When general standards of hygiene are low, such as is hard to avoid in homes for the mentally handicapped, the incidence of faecally-borne illness is high.

The hands should always be washed before eating, a habit which varies widely from country to country. In Portugal, for example, even simple roadside restaurants commonly have a handbasin outside, in which every customer washes his hands before going in to eat.

The effectiveness of handwashing is demonstrated by a story which was told by the Australian medical biologist and Nobel Laureate Sir Macfarlane Burnet. In 1954 a polio epidemic was in its early stages in Western Australia, and the State was due to be visited by Queen Elizabeth II. The polio virus is most commonly spread by excrement carried on the hands of children, and the dilemma facing the authorities was whether or not to take a highly unpopular step and forbid children to attend the festivities, as masses of them together could cause rapid spread and make the epidemic worse. The final decision was to allow children to attend the public gatherings, but to insist that families and teachers in charge of groups of children should make certain that every pair of hands was washed with soap and water after any visit to the toilet. Not only was there no flare-up of

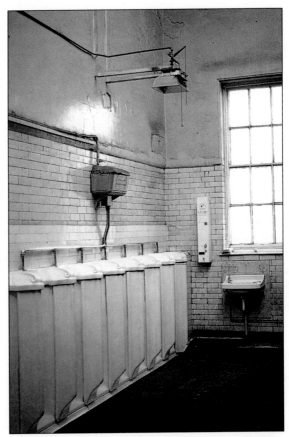

Figure 77   Diseases spread by the faecal-oral route would be greatly reduced if people were more careful about washing their hands.

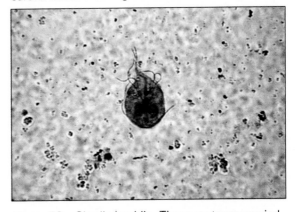

Figure 78   Giardia lamblia. These protozoa carried in the bowel and transmitted as cysts may infect food and are one of the most common causes of diarrhoea among children in the developing countries and frequently affect international travellers.

the epidemic, the incidence of new cases of polio actually fell during and immediately after the Queen's visit.

Some people have to take particular care with the washing of their hands, and of these the biggest group numerically are the cooks of the world, in family homes, restaurants and institutional kitchens. In well-run organisations training of personnel will stress the importance of this simple measure, but a simple instruction to 'wash your hands' will have little impact unless it is supported by explanation of the need for the edict and due emphasis is placed on its importance by management's attitude to related regulations and standard procedures. It is, for example, more important that the food is served with clean hands than it is to smile at the customer who is about to eat it.

In all kitchens, running water should be freely available for washing the hands frequently during the food preparation process, because fresh food may well be carrying organisms which cause illness if ingested. As always, after each wash, the hands should be thoroughly dried.

The organisms carried in the bowel which may go on to infect food include protozoa which may be transmitted in the form of cysts, including some that are quite common in Britain, such as *Giardia lamblia*, and in the tropics, the amoebae. Studies have shown that the commonest route of infection is from mother to children, then children to children, and then children to parents: a cycle which is easy enough to break, given sufficient attention to a simple countermeasure.

Those who are involved in the care of sick people have to pay particular attention to the washing of hands, and the removal of bacteria may need to be aided by antiseptic soaps in the case of surgeons, nurses, dentists and so on. Constant scrubbing may soften the skin, and normal do-it-yourself activities are liable to cause minor injury. This can be best avoided by the regular use of a moisturising hand cream during and after washing.

Any cuts or sores in the hands of food handlers and others who might pass on infection must be covered with wound dressings which are dark blue in colour. If the blue dressing falls into the food product it can then be spotted easily, and the contaminated food condemned.

Infections spread by the airborne route can be minimised if people take care to avoid the exposure of other people to their bacteria by way of spray from the nose or mouth, such as occurs when coughing, sneezing, laughing or talking.

The prettiest and friendliest pets may have recently been rooting around in a rubbish tip, and should be assumed to be carrying pathogenic bacteria. Reference to Chapter 6 will indicate several diseases which can be carried by animals, including pets, and a pet around the house should mean more frequent washing by everybody, especially where children are concerned. Strange animals should not be fondled. Dogs in the countryside are best not allowed into the house, and certainly not into the kitchen.

Simple measures of personal hygiene can be extremely effective in blocking the transmission of infection, to the extent that if they were universally adhered to, many infections would cease to spread. These are simple steps that all of us can take, as a personal contribution to infection control.

9

Global Control of Infectious Disease

Most present endeavours in infection control are centred on the protection of specific *communities* against diseases which may periodically erupt among them, by preventing entry of the diseases and transmission from person to person; and on the protection of *individuals* from diseases which are already endemic within those communities. It sometimes happens, however, that a disease is of such universally accepted importance, and has features which make such an approach a practical proposition, that *global* control is justified, even to the extent that total eradication may be envisaged.

Disease control is now accepted as being essentially a matter for the state, but it was not always that way. In days gone by, religious bodies and philanthropic institutions made the running by clearing jungles, sweeping roads, setting up sanatoria and asylums, and preaching against life-shortening abuse of the body such as heavy drinking. But individual initiative is not in itself enough to bring about great changes in society, and such activities awakened the conscience of those responsible for public administration. Thus, responsibility for change finally came to rest with public bodies so influential that they were in a position to improve living standards by the provision of services of a quality allowing a hygienic and dignified way of life.

'Public health', in the sense that the state accepts responsibility for activities designed to promote it, is quite a new concept. Even now, in some countries, the promotion of public health takes a lowly priority behind, for example, the promotion of war. It is hardly surprising that in these places health problems in the late twentieth century, including those of infectious disease, are roughly similar to those faced back in the Middle Ages by people of the now-developed world.

CONTROL AND ERADICATION

For a short time after the end of the second world war it must have seemed to many people that the complete eradication of infectious disease from the world was a practical possibility. The micro-organisms responsible for all the important diseases had been identified. Vaccines could prevent many of them, and those which were not preventable man was able, for the first time in two thousand years of study, to treat by killing the bacteria that were causing them. The vectors for 'most of the diseases carried by animals and arthropods were known, and also for the first time man had at his disposal powerful insecticidal chemicals that would not cause harm to human beings.

In particular geographical areas, indeed, whole diseases had already been wiped out. Towards the end of the nineteenth century and at the beginning of the twentieth, the end of yellow fever, smallpox, typhus and cholera in the American continent north of Mexico had been seen, and the end of the latter three in the British Isles and parts of continental Europe. Plague and malaria had essentially been eliminated from the advanced countries, and the diseases which caused most of the childhood deaths in the nineteenth century – dysentery, scarlet fever, and diphtheria – had become rare and usually mild. All of the major advances had taken place in the preceding 100 years, and some of the most spectacular only in the previous five, during the war years. Was there anything man could not do?

In this final chapter some aspects of the process by which infectious disease is managed at the global level are examined, and the prospects for the eradication of some of the great scourges of mankind are reviewed. Detailed mechanisms are now known for the prevention, treatment and control of spread of most of them, and several have been outlined in this book. Hence, the principles are known. It is translating these principles into practice that creates the difficulties, and the examples of smallpox and malaria are examined – one global campaign that succeeded in totally eradicating the disease, and one that failed – in order to see just what those difficulties are. We then go on to consider the lessons which such great global efforts may have for all of us in managing infection and infectious disease.

It was in this spirit of optimism that the WHO was founded, and set among its goals the complete eradication from the world, as a start, of the diseases malaria and smallpox, with others to follow.

Forty years later, it is still only smallpox that has been made totally extinct. Is that failure, or a triumph?

It might be as well at this point to clear up some semantic confusion. The purist view of 'eradication' is that the pathogen has been made extinct, that not one single example exists anywhere in the world. While admirably clear and precise, this definition makes it in practice impossible to plan for the eradication of any existing infectious disease. Others have used the term 'elimination' to express an aim somewhere short of complete eradication, with the disease still prevalent but at a low level, with the term 'control' meaning a level of prevalence rather higher again, but stable.

This is more than just playing with words, as there is an extremely important practical difference between eradicating a disease and controlling it. Controlling costs money, time and resources, whereas none of these resources need be expended on a disease which has been eradicated. Hence, in order to achieve eradication it might be worth while spending a lot for a comparatively short time, in order to avoid paying rather less each year, but for ever. Epidemiologists and health administrators are attracted to the idea of eradication, therefore, for strictly economic as well as for health reasons.

In practice, the concept of eradication is now almost entirely confined to *regional* rather than *global* application. Hence, eradication can be defined as the purposeful reduction of the prevalence of a disease to the point where no further transmission occurs, within a defined area, by means of a defined campaign, and limited in time.

What diseases, then, are among the candidates for eradication? There are several factors which need consideration in order to decide on the status of such candidacy, factors which have moderated some of the earlier enthusiasm with a readier appreciation of just what is practicable and what is not. The prospects for the eradication of a disease, on a local as well as a world scale, depend greatly on the ecological relationship of the infecting micro-organism with man and on the way the disease is transmitted. René Dubos, in *Man Adapting*, has suggested that on the basis of this relationship microbes can be divided broadly into two groups, exogenous pathogens and endogenous ones.

Organisms acquired from an exogenous source come from an infected person or animal. Exposure to these pathogens causes a specific and well-defined disease within a finite time (the incubation period). These organisms cannot survive for long in the environment free from their hosts, and tend not to fall into a commensal relationship with man or cause long-lasting, chronic infection. Diseases caused by this group include smallpox, malaria, typhus, yellow fever, and measles. They were until recently the major infections of concern everywhere, and remain so (with the exception of smallpox) in the developing countries.

Infections caused by the endogenous group are quite different. The organisms are commonly present in the human body, existing for example in the nose, throat or intestinal tract without causing harm. The clinical syndromes they cause are less easily defined than those caused by the exogenous group, and one organism may replace another during the course of an infection. Examples are urinary tract infections, wound infections, and even 'septicaemia' (or blood 'poisoning'), especially in hospitals, where endogenous organisms are the main cause of infection.

Some organisms, obviously, may fall into an intermediate category according to circumstances, and these include the salmonellae, streptococci and staphylococci with which we co-exist in what is sometimes rather an uneasy relationship. But the point of this classification is that it would be impossible ever to contemplate eradication of diseases, severe or otherwise, caused by organisms in the endogenous or intermediate groups. All these organisms are persistent survivors, and the illnesses they cause can be 'taken over' by replacements; further, they are capable of considerable antigenic shift.

It follows that eradication is only possible in the case of microbes falling into the exogenous category and the diseases they cause, whether on a large-scale local, a regional, or a global basis.

The next important factor is the extent to which man is the natural reservoir, as opposed to creatures in the animal world. All human infections have their animal counterparts, with the closeness of the relationship varying widely. In the case of the zoonoses, the micro-organisms causing the animal and the human diseases are identical, because the diseases are animal diseases which are normally transmitted from animal to animal, with man becoming infected only accidentally; examples include plague, rabies and brucellosis. Eradication depends entirely on the feasibility of eradication within the animal reservoir, taking into account the ruthlessness with which we are prepared to go about destroying infected wildlife and domestic stock. On a regional basis, it can be done: Britain eradicated rabies, and brucellosis has been eradicated in the United States. Aided by quarantine and port controls, plague has just about

been eradicated in the developed world. But few other zoonoses are worth the resources it would take to eradicate them, and to eradicate infections among most forms of wildlife (jungle yellow fever, scrub typhus, or psittacosis, for example) would be impossible, short of extermination of several entire species. The theoretical possibility exists that if a human disease (say, smallpox) is eliminated then a related animal disease (say, cowpox or monkeypox) will march in and replace it, but this does not seem ever to have happened in practice.

The mode of transmission is another factor which will affect the chance of eradication. In the case of faecal-oral spread, as we commented earlier, if a substantial dose of the organism is required in order to cause illness, then control is feasible in areas with a high level of sanitation, but complete eradication is inconceivable, even in the best managed environments. When viruses are the infecting agents, the problem is even harder to tackle.

Droplet-spread infections can be eradicated by widespread immunisation if only single, specific antigens are involved, and if infection or immunisation brings about solid immunity. Universal immunisation in infancy can cause the complete disappearance of an organism. However, when the organisms are of many and variable antigenic types, with influenza being the notorious example, eradication is not possible. Also, if the infection is a very long-lasting one – the chickenpox virus, for example, can rest for years in the body and emerge years later as shingles – this again rules out eradication.

Diseases *spread by biting vectors* can be eradicated from urban areas, and if the only reservoir is human, as in the case of malaria, wider-scale eradication can be envisaged. The success of eradication measures depends, as we will see, on human rather than biological factors.

As we suggested in the section dealing with the control of the diseases *spread by contact*, eradication – athough possible in principle – is not in practice likely to be possible by measures which would be acceptable to the public in a democratic society.

When eradication is to be attempted, the mechanisms are basically those already described in this book, with modifications only of scale. The chain of transmission must be broken, and for eradication to be practicable there should be one main control measure which is completely effective, simple in application and comparatively inexpensive. Where appropriate, the entry of pathogens should be prevented by quarantine. Susceptible individuals should be protected, the best method being by immunisation in childhood, and in default of that, measures employed which prevent the organisms entering by their usual portal or which destroy them before they can set up the infective process. And, very importantly, the epidemiological features of the disease should allow surveillance and detection of the rare cases which will occur in the later stages of the programme.

Other preconditions for eradication fall into social and economic categories rather than technical. The disease must be recognised as being of sufficient importance to warrant the effort which will be expended, and there must be some reason why eradication is a better option than continuing control. And it follows, naturally, that the necessary resources must be available.

The evolution of approaches to eradication of a disease has led the WHO to define approaches in four phases.

First there is the *preparatory phase*, including the training of personnel, taking necessary censuses and setting up the administrative structure. The *'attack' phase* follows, with the chosen control measure employed over the whole area, the aim being to stop transmission as quickly as possible and continue until human infections have died out. In the case of malaria, for example, it takes a year to stop transmission, and then another three years until all parasites are cleared from the population.

When the prevalence has reached a previously-agreed low level, the *consolidation phase* and epidemiological surveillance begin, involving surveys of morbidity, study of continuing laboratory data, and the detection and reporting of remaining individual cases. Obtaining such data is only necessary when eradication is the objective, and new methods have had to be established in order that it is done thoroughly.

The *maintenance phase* starts when eradication has been successful, and lasts as long as the infection is to be found anywhere in the world. Administration of this phase is usually a task for the health services of the country concerned, but if these services are not capable of the necessary level of vigilance, then planning for the maintenance phase has to be included in the overall plan. Any

new cases must be picked up quickly, and laboratory supported diagnosis must be fast, which predicates a given minimum level of health service technology.

THE ERADICATION OF SMALLPOX

Smallpox was known in ancient times in the east, and it possibly entered Europe with the marauding invaders. It affects the whole body, including causing eruptions of the skin which are very similar to those of chickenpox. After healing, the lesions leave pockmarks. It existed in epidemic form in England in the seventeenth century, affecting royalty no less than the poor, and from the continent of Europe it was transported to Mexico and the rest of the New World, where it had a devastating impact. Most of the Spanish and other invaders were immune, but the infection was new to the Americas and caused terrible epidemics among the Indian people.

Vaccination proved to be a highly effective means of controlling smallpox in both the Old and the New World, but the disease was still prevalent well into the twentieth century. As recently as 1930, England and Wales recorded 12,000 cases of smallpox, and in the United States over 48,000 cases were seen. However, by the end of the 1940s in the continents of North America and Europe the disease was no longer endemic. But in several countries it was indeed still endemic, and a high degree of diligence in the surveillance, case detection and containment of outbreaks was required to hold the global situation constant. Children were immunised as a routine in the developed countries, and the smallpox vaccination certificate was a virtually universal requirement for travellers.

In 1959 the World Health Assembly passed a resolution calling for the global eradication of smallpox by means of intense campaigns of immunisation in those places where the disease was still endemic. It was pointed out that more was being spent on controlling smallpox than would be needed to eradicate it, but in the following seven years there was virtually no progress in the endemic areas. National initiative was lacking, resources were not being applied, and the vaccine was insufficiently potent by the time it was used. So, in 1966, with smallpox still endemic in more than 30 countries, the World Health Assembly decided to intensify the global programme, with the declared objective being eradication by 1976. A special budget was allocated, and a new unit was established at WHO headquarters.

The aim of the attack phase was systematically to vaccinate entire populations wherever fewer than 80% had been immunised previously. The phase would be deemed to have ended when the incidence of the disease was less than five cases a year for each 100,000 population, and where about 80% of the population were immunised.

In the consolidation phase every new case was followed up and contacts traced, with intensive local immunisation where cases occurred. New babies were all vaccinated. Each of these two phases was estimated to require two years, so for each national programme the minimum time would be four years. Final certification was to be by the WHO with the aid of an independent international panel.

When the campaign started, there were major reservoirs of the disease in central Asia, Africa south of the Sahara, Indonesia and Brazil. The campaign was vigorous from the very beginning, with a high priority placed on the supply of adequate quantities of high-quality vaccine. By 1970 all countries had sufficient supplies, and high-pressure jet injectors were introduced in order to speed the procedure. These proved impractical, however, in the deep countryside and where skilled technicians were not available, and a cheap, simple and highly satisfactory replacement was the double-pronged needle. A small drop of vaccine clings between the prongs, and a number of quick pricks completes the procedure. Studies showed that there was a benefit in terms of subsequent infection in cleaning the skin beforehand with alcohol or any other fluid, and the resulting speed of the whole process was an important benefit in itself.

Within a single year there was a marked trend towards a lower incidence, despite a far higher level of reliable notification, with the fastest drops being in central and west Africa. By 1972, local cases of smallpox were still occurring in only eight of the originally endemic countries, and South America was free from the disease. In Africa, smallpox was confined to Botswana, Ethiopia and the Sudan, and in Asia the endemic area extended from Bangladesh through northern India and Nepal to Pakistan.

But the remaining difficulties were daunting. The campaign had only got started in Ethiopia as late as 1971. In Sudan, the area where smallpox was still occurring was in a state of civil war. In Bangladesh, a resurgence of the disease had coincided with political upheavals and the return of refugees from a crowded refugee camp near Calcutta. As the campaign neared its global goal, therefore, the frustrating fact was that the remaining areas were the ones wracked by civil disturbance and breakdown in social order. The focus had to remain on Asia and east Africa.

In northern India, the problem was surveillance, and a massive village-to-village, and later house-to-house, search was undertaken for smallpox cases. This led to an enormous apparent increase in the incidence of the disease, with cries of dismay about the 'failure' of the programme among the public and in the press. In Bangladesh, there were enormous difficulties tracking refugees from flood-devastated areas, with people moving in their hundreds of thousands across drowned lowlands, many of them in a highly infectious state. Despite all this, a final outbreak was brought under control, and the last case in Asia was that of a little girl in 1975.

In east Africa, the cease-fire in the Sudan enabled freeing of that country from smallpox by the end of 1972, but Ethiopia remained a serious obstacle to final success. As the programme at last swung into action in that country in 1971, 26,000 cases were identified by the search teams, and mass vaccination brought this down to 4400 in 1974. But these were in appalling areas to try to achieve anything: one was in the desolate Ogaden desert in the south, and the other in the mountainous countryside of the north, one of the hardest places to reach in the whole of Africa. Further, the local people were vigorously opposed to modern techniques of immunisation; they practised variolation with the live virus, and it took months of patient negotiation before they would allow themselves to be vaccinated. In addition to surveillance, special searches were made of places where smallpox sufferers might be hidden.

Outbreaks occurred in 1977 in Somalia and Kenya, and in those countries, too, intensive surveillance was established and the outbreaks contained. By the end of that year, the disease was not being transmitted anywhere in the world, and many countries had ceased the routine vaccination of children. Ethiopia, Somalia and Kenya were

Figure 79 In a wonderful achievement, the World Health Organisation has overseen the complete elimination of smallpox, one of the most feared diseases of all time.

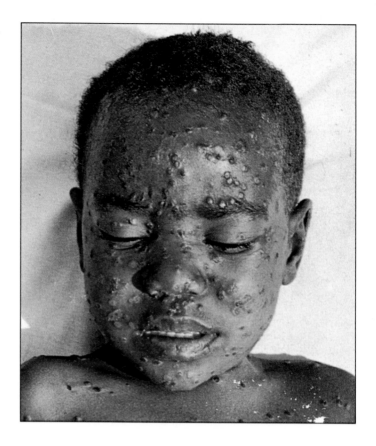

certified as being free from smallpox in October 1979, no cases having been identified since the last one, a hospital cook in Merka, Somalia, in October 1977.

This was not, as it turned out, to be the last case of smallpox in history. That doubtful honour goes to the mother of a medical photographer at the University of Birmingham, who had been working on the floor above a laboratory where the smallpox virus was being studied, became infected with smallpox, and died. Her mother was also diagnosed as having the disease, but eventually recovered. Now, the only two existing samples of the virus are kept under high security at laboratories in Atlanta, Georgia, and in Moscow.

The objective of eradicating endemic smallpox from the globe had been achieved. What, then, were the factors that made it possible for mankind deliberately to eradicate a major infectious disease from the face of the earth, for the first time in history?

The condition that there should be a cheap and

effective single control measure was fulfilled from the start. Further, case detection and surveillance were aided by the obvious rash and lesions of the active disease, and by the scars left by old disease and vaccination.

However, the situation in regard to resources and organisation at the outset was so poor that it is a wonder the campaign ever got started. In fact, the campaign was always short of funds, but some of the richest and most powerful countries supported it, and it was provided with inspiring leadership from the WHO and the chief of its Smallpox Eradication Programme, Dr Donald Henderson. Quite apart from smallpox, the campaign administrators had to deal at various times with a political crisis in East Pakistan/Bangladesh and the resulting flood of refugees, the war between Somalia and Ethiopia and the continuing civil war in the latter, civil wars in Sudan and Nigeria, and 17 minor coups in 18 west African countries participating in the campaign!

Although the countries from which it was finally

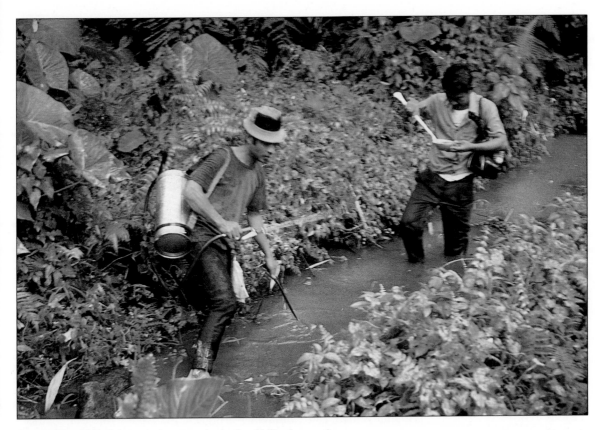

Figure 80 Malarial control measures in the Philippines using chemical sprays.

eradicated were the ones least able to help themselves, assistance from other countries could be justified in the light of enlightened self-interest. When the cost of the campaign for the ten-year period 1967–76 was tabulated, the WHO found that 83 million dollars had been contributed by international assistance and about twice that amount by the governments of the countries where the disease was not endemic. The estimated annual cost to countries where the disease was not endemic had been one to two billion dollars in quarantine and immunisation measures, none of which would be further required.

THE MALARIA ERADICATION CAMPAIGN

The campaign against malaria started before the smallpox campaign, and was the first international eradication programme to be undertaken on a wholly global scale. When the role of the mosquito was discovered towards the end of the nineteenth century, malaria control measures were mainly directed against the larval stage of the vector, by physical elimination of the watery breeding grounds, killing them with oil and other chemicals, and by changing the ecology of the environment. These measures worked well in urban and rural areas with dense populations.

The introduction in the 1940s of DDT and other cheap and highly effective insecticides revolutionised the whole approach to vector control. Spraying the walls of houses is much cheaper and easier than changing the physical structure of the whole environment. For the first time, because spraying of individual houses would protect those who lived in them, prevention of malaria in rural areas became a feasible proposition.

Early results with house spraying were dramatic,

with transmission being totally prevented even in highly malarious areas of the world, such as southern Italy, Greece, and some parts of South America and South-East Asia. In Greece, spraying was discontinued in 1952 because of shortage of money, but it was then found that the occurrence was at such a low level that surveillance and treatment of individual cases were sufficient to prevent transmission recurring.

It was in Greece, too, that the first signs of resistance of the anopheles mosquito to DDT began to appear. Three pressures, then, arose to stimulate moves towards deliberate eradication of malaria world wide during a finite period: a cheap and effective measure was available to stop transmission; the measure was threatening to lose its effectiveness through resistance if continued indefinitely; and (as was later shown for smallpox) continuing 'control' measures were in the long run going to cost more than a concentrated effort on eradication.

Further, malaria has a severely debilitating effect and makes labour less effective through premature death and loss of working time because of sickness. Chronically affected farmers were being robbed of initiative, and to eradicate malaria would assist subsistence farming populations to break out of the vicious cycle of poverty, malnutrition and primitive farming.

Accordingly, in 1955 the World Health Assembly resolved that one of the main objectives of the WHO should be the world-wide eradication of malaria, with the rashly optimistic statement that this could be attained within five years.

The basis of the strategy was to be the four phases outlined in the above description of the smallpox campaign, except that the preparatory and attack phases were to a large extent combined. This was because of the control measure chosen, spraying the interior surfaces of houses. To be effective, every house had to be sprayed, and therefore as part of the preparatory process a census was needed to establish just where every house was. The insecticides chosen were DDT and HCH (benzene hexachloride) and the chemically-related dieldrin. All had a good residual effect when sprayed on walls in the proper amount, remained lethal for about six months, and were relatively cheap.

The reason why these interior residual sprays were so effective has to do with the habits of the mosquito and the life cycle of the malaria parasite.

The time between the mosquito feeding on infected blood and being able to transmit the infection is around ten days. The mosquito feeds about every two or three days, and after feeding normally rests on an interior surface. This means that after taking a meal of infected blood, the mosquito will go to rest on a lethally poisonous surface some three times before it can pass on the infection, so the chances are it will be killed before it has a chance to do so.

Spraying all dwellings should interrupt transmission totally within eighteen months, and has to be continued for another three years so that all existing human infections can be cured while transmission continues to be prevented. Latterly, of course, surveillance becomes the most important activity, and this is one aspect of malaria eradication where it was at a substantial disadvantage compared to smallpox, because the existence of infection can only be confirmed by inspection of the blood under the microscope. The clinical features are too vague for definite diagnosis, or may be lacking altogether. 'Fever', which is a symptom most sufferers will show at some time or another, was used as a basic screening identifier, and the detection of cases involved canvassing all houses for cases of fever and obtaining samples of blood for examination. Vigilance, which is the motivation and capacity to carry out this often thankless and tiring work, was to prove one of the downfalls of the campaign, and by the end of 1960 it was apparent that not enough planning had gone into this aspect at the outset.

At the start, the response of most countries to the eradication programme appeared to be highly encouraging, and by the end of 1958, 63 countries had either initiated eradication programmes or converted existing 'control' programmes to eradication. In 1962 a peak was reached, with 65 countries (737 million people) in operational phases.

But causes for serious concern were appearing. In spite of efficiently conducted spraying operations, in some areas transmission was persisting and this appeared to be not only because the mosquitoes were becoming physiologically resistant to the insecticides but also because they were refusing to cooperate with the campaign. The mosquitoes maintaining transmission of malaria were not resting on the sprayed internal walls but flying from the dwellings and resting outside, apparently to some extent because the insecticides were hurting their feet. The characteristics of some of the anopheles species which had made them efficient vectors were also those that made them vulnerable to interior spraying, but other species, with predominantly 'refractory' outdoor resting and biting habits, became the main causes of persistent transmission in the so-called 'problem' areas. The species *Anopheles albimanus* is an example of a 'bite-and-run' mosquito, as they were dubbed, because they would bite indoors and fly outside, unharmed by the insecticide. In Central America, this species is the principal vector of malaria. Also, in some areas the people – especially during periods of migration – were sleeping outside and were getting bitten in the open air, or they were living in makeshift dwellings with such insubstantial walls that if they were sprayed at all, there was insufficient surface to absorb an adequate dose.

In 1966, the campaign was reviewed by the WHO Expert Committee on Malaria. A survey in 1960 had reported optimistically that 73% of the programmes had good prospects for success, with 20% being doubtful and none unfavourable. In 1966, however, a repeat study indicated that *only* 29% were now regarded as having good prospects, 52% doubtful and 19% unfavourable. It was concluded that the outstanding factor affecting the prospect of a favourable outcome was adequate planning and financing of surveillance operations, and member states of the WHO, facing in many cases severe financial problems, called for re-examination of the whole global strategy.

One of the main reasons that some countries were finding the eradication programme hard to finance, even with assistance, was that they had grossly underestimated the extent of the resource commitment which would be required. The original estimate of the planners was that necessary programmes could be financed at a level compatible with even simple economies if the eradication could be completed within a limited time. However, programmes running well over time were not only ineffective, they were very expensive to maintain. Some countries, too, had agreed to join in the global campaign in a precipitate and unplanned manner, because the official international policy – agreed upon by the WHO and other major health aid agencies – was that only eradication programmes would be eligible for outside support. Consequently many control programmes were converted to eradication

in name alone, with no prospect of success.

Technically, it was by this time clear that the inside spraying of dwellings which had been so successful in urban and stable rural communities was far less effective when life styles were characterised by scattered and migratory patterns, with habitation in huts and temporary shelters. Effective spraying was in theory possible even in these areas, but required a level of skill and individual initiative from the men doing the spraying that was unobtainable in the areas in question. Although the affected populations might have been small, malaria among them was readily transmitted to surrounding villages and towns.

Surveillance, with strict attention paid to the detection of individual cases and to regular timed follow-ups, had not been realised by most countries to be such a burden, and supervision of proper treatment was also harder than had been expected.

The conclusion of the global review of strategy was that where malaria was still a concern and a threat, but eradication deemed to be impossible, then an unpalatable alternative course would have to be taken: namely, reversion from eradication to control. This was an unpalatable option because the ultimate benefits of eradication would have to be foregone, and at little or no saving to the country's budget. Antimalarial measures would be diversified to meet local circumstances, instead of relying almost entirely on spraying inside dwellings with residual insecticides.

A whole new set of nationally planned control programmes were established after 1969, to the benefit especially of several countries in Africa, in some of which there had been no programme beforehand of any kind. Some other governments faced a real dilemma in deciding whether to convert from eradication to control, or to carry through the existing eradication programme, and balancing the costs and benefits was a tricky calculation. In many parts of Asia progress stopped after 1969, and in South-East Asia the number of reported cases of malaria began to rise alarmingly.

Compounding the problem was the phasing out of aid by the biggest international agencies, in particular the United Nations Children's Fund (UNICEF) and the US Agency for International Development, which had been prepared to support eradication programmes with a defined end to them, but not control programmes with an open-ended commitment when there were so many other pressing health problems also deserving support.

The present situation is that while there is reasonable hope for steady improvement of malaria control by the sort of diversified activities we discussed in the last chapter, there is little chance of further gains in the eradication of malaria in the foreseeable future. The refractory behaviour of mosquitoes was compounded by an increasing problem of resistance to insecticides. In Europe, resistance did not develop fast enough to prevent eradication; but in warmer climates, vectors were becoming resistant to both DDT and dieldrin, and some species had meanwhile also become resistant to replacement insecticides which were already being used for pest control in agriculture.

The eradication programme did have its successes. In the temperate climatic zones, where most of the developed countries with originally malarious areas are situated, malaria was eradicated during the global campaign, and the whole of Europe was freed from malaria, together with coastal areas (where most people live) in South America. In the tropical zones, eradication was mainly successful in the islands, notably the Caribbean, where compactly defined territory combined with a degree of isolation made management of the campaign easier, particularly during the later stages when tight surveillance was

required. There were a few individually astonishing successes; in Taiwan, for example, among a population of 13 million people, there were a million cases in 1954 and nine in 1969.

The global malaria eradication programme broke down basically because it could not move fast enough, for a wide range of organisational, practical, economic and political reasons. The WHO foresaw the problem with vector resistance, one of the main reasons for embarking on an eradication programme in the first place, but resistance continued to develop too fast for lagging national programmes. Replacements for DDT were ecologically unacceptable or too expensive, or already ineffective because of resistance. The refractory behaviour of mosquito species had not been foreseen. Accordingly, the factor which is essential for the success of any global eradication campaign, the availability of a single, simple and cheap measure for breaking the transmission chain, after only a few years had ceased to exist.

THE MAINTENANCE OF INFECTION CONTROL

Several themes have recurred throughout this book, embracing all aspects of infection control and ranging from the importance of individual pathogens and illnesses to the sweep of history and

Figure 81 Village in Zimbabwe where a carefully designed latrine is under construction to reduce the spread of infection from faeces.

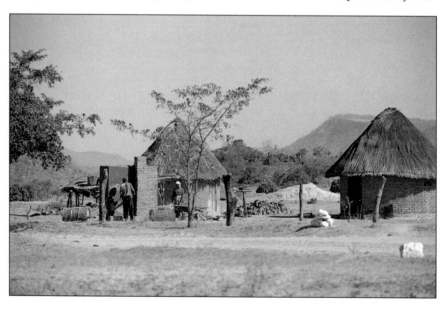

international efforts to wipe out diseases from the globe. They are of universal significance, and relate to individual human behaviour as well as to the behaviour of institutions and governments. They concern the way that systems of infection control are managed and maintained, and have little directly to do with medical diagnosis and treatment. Many lessons of direct relevance to man have emerged from global efforts at infection control, such as the examples described above, and in this section some of these lessons are reviewed.

Organisation

Organisation is as important to the control of infection within a home, a hospital or a restaurant as it is for a national government which decides to attempt to eradicate an endemic disease from an entire region.

A poorly-organised structure for the systematic delivery of health care to all that need it, especially at primary-care levels and in rural areas, means that much existing knowledge about the control of infectious disease will not be used. This is now the case in many developing countries. Further, there are substantial differences in approach across shared international borders, and it is not uncommon for people in one place to die from infectious diseases which could be prevented or successfully treated in another place only a few miles away.

The global malaria eradication programme started going wrong because some administrations had not planned how to undertake the tasks involved, and were poorly organised to administer them when they were running. In different spheres of human activity, exactly the same principles apply. An institutional kitchen, restaurant or roadside fast-food outlet would be presumed to have among its goals the supply of food which does not poison any of its clients. But even if the managers and supervisors know all the microbiology in the world, this is of no value if individual food handlers do not understand how they also fit into the scheme of things, and if things are not so organised that the capacity of individual staff for infecting food is at a minimum. At home, domestic affairs can be organised in such a way that the risk of infection from food or droplets is minimised and, when it does occur, that the risk of others becoming infected within or outside the home is minimal.

Surveillance

Surveillance is a matter which has been mentioned on several occasions, because it is the key to monitoring the control of infectious disease on a national or international level.

Surveillance is a term which used to be applied in a limited sense to observation of sick individuals and their contacts, but it now refers to the continuing scrutiny of all aspects of occurrence and spread of infection which could affect the effectiveness of control within whole populations. The modern approach to surveillance includes the systematic collection and arrangement of data, and the prompt dissemination of information to those who can make effective use of it. Methods of surveillance will have advantages and disadvantages depending on the disease to be surveyed, but will include:

- routine reports from hospitals and individual health workers of deaths and non-fatal diseases;

- special investigations of outbreaks of disease;

- identification in the laboratory of infective agents;

- information on the use, effectiveness and side effects of vaccines and antibacterial drugs;

- information on the proportion of people in populations who are immune to particular diseases.

It is a matter of judgement as to which infections need controlling in particular circumstances, and so, although it is neither possible nor necessary to maintain full surveillance of all infections at all times, it is necessary to collect enough information to enable decisions to be made on how control resources should be allocated. Most nations have regulations which make it mandatory for doctors to report the occurrence of certain illnesses to the authorities. This can be a reliable process for dramatic and rare conditions, but it is exceedingly unreliable for most of the common diseases we could come across any day, and is completely inadequate for the provision of early warning of new epidemics and 'new' illnesses. Such regulations do allow some monitoring of changes in incidence over periods of time, but an example of the weakness of a reporting system is that it only takes a single but well-publicised expression of great interest and concern in a particular disease for it then to be notified with unprecedented assiduity. Rare or otherwise, its incidence thus quite falsely appears to rocket upward, and this may lead to pressures for quite possibly unjustified diversion of resources to its control.

In the developed countries there are now systems whereby results from laboratories are referred to central reference centres for collation. In Britain, for example, it is the Communicable Diseases Surveillance Centre which is the focal point, and the collated information is published in the form of regular *Communicable Disease Reports*, distributed all over the country. At US Federal Government level, the Centers for Disease Control have a similar function, and publish the *Morbidity and Mortality Weekly Reports*. At international level, the WHO monitors infectious disease in the ways referred to earlier; that of tracking the course of influenza is the one which is of most direct interest to most people.

Again, there are clear lessons to be learnt at the local, institutional and personal levels. The housekeeper can be constantly on the lookout for sources of infection, and be on the alert for signs of it among the family. The manager of an institution can keep not only accurate records and statistics, but also a personal eye open for adherence to procedural rules and requirements affecting, for example, the handling of food. In hospitals, most already have systems for monitoring outbreaks of infection, and more subtle monitors include the recording of rates of infection associated with the work of particular surgeons, teams, and units.

Present-day surveillance methods provide good information on the prevalence and incidence of disease, allow the identification of places and people that are at high risk, allow recognition at the earliest possible time of increases in incidence and the outbreak of epidemics, and encourage effective monitoring and evaluation of control activities. Modern techniques of surveillance are now being applied to a wide range of environmental problems and hazards and, in relation to infectious disease, they have largely superseded old systems of epidemiological evaluation and obsolete quarantine regulations and procedures.

Environmental management

Environmental management is the key to easing reliance on the vagaries of human behaviour. If a thing cannot be done wrongly, it will not be; but, as we all know, if a thing can be done wrongly, sooner or later it will be. Environmental management ranges from the filling and draining of whole areas so that mosquitoes cannot breed, through the supply of clean and pure water piped directly to homes, to the processing of milk and other food and the use of screens at home to prevent disease-carrying vectors alighting on people or their food.

Quarantine and containment

Quarantine and containment of infectious disease are necessary when all else has failed, and existing disease must be blocked off where it stands. In the case of rabies, for example, rigorous quarantine measures limit the access to the shores of rabies-free countries such as Britain and Australia of animals which just could be carrying the disease. The risk may be small, but the consequences for domestic stock and wildlife are so horrendous that only the lowest attainable risk is acceptable. However, the use of quarantine has declined substantially with improvements in the scale and analytical ability of surveillance measures, as well as improvements in other infection control measures and an increased understanding of the natural history of disease. Quarantine means limitation of freedom for people and animals who are well, but who have been exposed to the possibility of infection. The period of quarantine will be at least as long as the longest possible incubation time of the disease and, if disease does occur, the method of quarantine will prevent further transmission to those who might be susceptible. The strictness of quarantine will depend on the disease, and may extend from keeping children away from school to complete isolation within restricted boundaries.

In some cases of infectious disease, individual clinicians will have to decide on the extent to which the sufferers must be kept away from others, with decisions ranging from what to do with the child with rubella to advice for the traveller newly returned from overseas with an unexplained fever. Isolation of individual patients, and 'barrier' nursing, may still be required for some.

On a global scale, international surveillance of diseases and their trends has largely replaced quarantine, some 600 years after the Venetians first required visiting ships to anchor offshore for forty days and nights.

Education and training

Education is a vital feature of infection control, especially for diseases hard to cope with at the community level in any other way. Efforts to control the spread of AIDS are a prominent contemporary example, but this is a disease with dramatic impact of global import. There is a great need for the same principles to be applied for the control of less dramatic infections. Although professionals in the health field are generally aware of methods for the control and treatment of infectious disease, they have been slow to share this knowledge with other people in an accessible form. Such sharing is best driven by a passionate belief in the virtues of education.

Education may be directed to a wide variety of groups, ranging from health professionals to members of the general public, and may be channelled through a wide variety of routes. It has a long history of endeavour, a patchy history of success, and a vast literature of its own. Health education is the process by which individuals and groups of people learn to promote, maintain or restore health. Most people cease being exposed to any formal efforts at health education once they leave school, so that new information is absorbed unsystematically from the newspapers, magazines, radio and television, information which may be correct or incorrect, partial or impartial, unbiased or biased.

Education for health must be directed at people as they are, with whatever interest they have or have not in improving their health and living conditions. Health education is easily derided, because efforts to develop a sense of responsibility for conditions of health are sometimes associated with a puritanical earnestness which is at odds with the lifestyle and aspirations of the target audience.

In the control of communicable disease, health education to be effective will have to be preceded by an appraisal of the community's existing level of knowledge about infection, together with assessment of existing habits and attitudes. Community health education programmes can then be designed to:

- change life styles, so that people become less susceptible to disease;
- change personal habits, so that disease is less likely to be transmitted from person to person;
- increase knowledge, so that people can assess without panic reports of outbreaks of disease and side effects of vaccines and antibacterial drugs, and make best use of preventive endeavours such as immunisation programmes.

Health education programmes can be designed for specific groups. New parents, for example, should obtain information on immunisation and hygienic baby care from doctors, clinics and community organisations. Trainee food handlers and catering staff will require special instruction on the preparation, preservation and handling of food. Farm workers need information on the safe handling of livestock and, especially in the developing countries, on the growing of agricultural products without adding to the risk of infection.

The best way of imparting all this information depends entirely on what it is and to whom it is addressed. Whatever the media employed, the credibility of the educators is of fundamental importance. For example, adamant official denials that a problem of any sort exists, say, with an antibacterial drug will be widely disdained when it becomes only too clear that there is a problem, albeit a tiny one which is easily outweighed by the benefits of the drug. But by the time people are being told about such benefits, all they can remember are the failures. The provision of accurate and reliable information to media communicators is an important and all-too-neglected part of health education.

INFECTION CONTROL AND THE FUTURE

In Britain and the rest of the developed world, the extent of success in combating infectious disease is manifest in the way that infection is no longer a subject of awe, let alone fear. Life expectancies are rising because of the longer survival of the newborn and the young, and other conditions have

Figure 82   Health education programmes in Uganda. New parents should be provided with information on immunisation and hygienic baby care from doctors, clinics and community organisations.

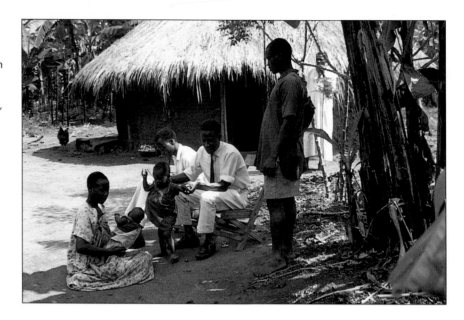

taken over as the commonest killers. The relative proportion of the elderly is increasing, forcing a whole set of new priorities on hard-pressed health resources.

Man has under control for the present at least the great epidemic diseases of the past, although only smallpox has been totally eradicated. Typhus and yellow fever are confined to defined areas, and although both cholera and plague continue to smoulder, they do so to a limited and controllable extent. Typhoid is rarely seen where the water is clean. Good control has also been gained of many of the diseases of childhood, such as diphtheria, poliomyelitis, whooping cough and measles, and tuberculosis is no longer the terror it was.

But we must not let infection lie unheeded, or turn our back on the threat it can still pose. The future holds many challenges, including the continually changing nature of infection, the movements of disease across national borders, the developing resistance of bacteria to drugs intended to kill them, and the lack of organisation and determination to combat infection on a large scale.

Whatever the advances in infection control over recent years, fever, famine and war remain the main threats to the health of mankind, and the stability of human communities. Infectious disease is far from being under control in the world as a whole. Malaria, one of the most important diseases of all time, has been checked in many places but is staging a strong comeback in others. Undramatic but lethal illnesses such as infant diarrhoea, with their spread fuelled by squalid living conditions, continue almost unabated. Influenza and other virus diseases which have recently become a threat are unchallenged at present by any generally useful therapeutic medicine. Vectors carrying disease are themselves becoming resistant to chemicals intended to destroy them.

These are threats which are immediately apparent to those living in the developing countries. But we all live in the same global village. No country is such an isolated unit that infectious disease within its borders can be so confined that there is no chance whatsoever that it could move to other nations, along with immigrants, workers, travellers, and all those who use the freedom of communication which has opened up the world over the last 50 years or so.

Therefore, while the future of infection control is a little different in the developing and the developed countries, all people face basically the same difficulties.

The most dramatic effect of disease control in general, and infection control in particular, has been its effect on population levels. Population growth has not been evenly distributed, but has affected – and will probably continue to affect – the poorer societies to a greater extent than the rich. Cities will probably continue to grow at a greater rate than rural areas, putting greater stress on water supplies and sewerage facilities and increasing the likelihood of spread of the diseases of overcrowding.

Infection control, of course, has not been the only cause of burgeoning populations. An accelerating trend in population growth was first apparent during the seventeenth and eighteenth centuries, and is commonly attributed to the industrial revolution. Another increase in the nineteenth century is likely to have been caused by the rise in living standards that became apparent during that time. The rate of growth rose more quickly in the first half of the present century, along with technological achievements and a continually rising standard of living. None of these rises can *primarily* have been the result of infection control but, as has been described, an important consequence of improvements in living standards and sanitation is the limitation of infectious disease.

However, since the second world war there has been a much faster rise in population than ever before, and to a large extent this must be attributable to controls in infectious disease brought about by the availability of modern drugs, the effectiveness of treatment and prevention, and the flow of this technology to the poorer parts of the world. General medical services have now made available to those who have never previously had them a vast array of preventive procedures, particularly effective in preventing the diseases of children, and increases in population among the young have had a flow-on effect in increased general fertility and a continuing accelerating growth in total numbers.

Some of the most startling increases in population have been in well-defined communities which have successfully tackled malaria, the best examples being Sri Lanka, Mauritius and British Guyana. Within a year of starting DDT spraying, crude mortalities in all three countries dropped sharply, infant mortality fell, birth rates rose, and populations soared. Again, of course, general medical services played their part in bringing about this effect; but in all countries where malaria has been brought under control, even when not eliminated, there have been impressive reductions in death rates. The effect of these campaigns, of course, is that in many places a newly pre-eminent priority is not the control of rates of infectious disease, it is the control of birth rates, with birth control being as essential as infection control.

Man will inevitably continue to see in the future more changes in the pattern of infectious disease of the kind outlined in Chapter 3. It is unlikely that we have seen the last of the 'new' dramatic infections imported in small numbers from exotic places, as were the Lassa and Ebola fevers and Marburg disease, but it is very improbable that they will ever pose a threat to whole communities in the developed world. A more realistic menace is antigenic change in the organisms causing diseases with which we are already very familiar and, of these, influenza will continue to be a threatening illness until a therapeutic drug is developed to combat it. Another example is cholera, which has changed its nature from the classic Asian type to a type known as 'El Tor', the bull, well established now in Africa and periodically ranging the world. The salmonella bacteria which so regularly appear in our food also have a remarkable capacity for change, and new strains are appearing in new sources, such as the meat of turkeys. It is possible that some organisms, previously only affecting animals, have the capacity to change their characteristics in such a way as to become pathogens for man – even AIDS may be part of this particular scenario.

Epidemiological surveillance will continue to be the most important single measure for quickly identifying and bringing under control new outbreaks of disease before they can take hold of whole populations.

Human activities will continue to make pathogens out of bacteria which might never have troubled us if we did not constantly make changes to our environment. For example, as air conditioning is increasingly used to improve living and working conditions, the possibility of infection by bacteria which live in air-conditioning units is increased, with *Legionella pneumophila* being the famous case in point. As personal and sexual behaviour changes, so does the threat from bacteria such as *Chlamydia* in causing urinary and pelvic infections. Crowding, eating on the run and other features of a busy urban life will maintain the transmission of respiratory and intestinal diseases, and as human behaviour patterns change, so too will the behaviour of pathogenic organisms.

It is inevitable that man will continue to discover that infection is at least one of the factors in inducing diseases for which he has previously not known the cause. This is especially likely to be so for many neurological conditions, as well as many of the cancerous diseases of the blood and bone-marrow systems.

In the laboratories and research centres, work will continue on immunisation, perhaps the most promising route of all for the continuing successful control of many of the worst diseases. Research will of course also continue on antibacterial drugs, but it is likely that improvements will be found in the refinement and continuing development of existing antibacterials rather than in the dramatic emergence of completely new categories of medicine.

The main problem facing the use of antibacterial drugs is that bacteria are developing resistance to them and, quite apart from the development of new products to overcome such resistance, a great deal of discipline will have to be maintained in the use of the existing ones. The human body, especially when young, has a remarkable capacity to cope with infection unaided by any antibiotics at all, and it will be as well that potential patients come to understand that antibiotics are not required simply because of the presence of infection. Resistance to antiobiotics in hospitals will continue to be a real problem, and increasingly refined and strict procedures will be needed to keep it under control.

Research into drugs for the treatment of diseases caused by viruses is still a wide open field, and it is here that we are likely to see the most spectacular advances in coming years. Vaccines are unlikely to be of as much practical use as antiviral drugs for treatment, because such a wide spectrum of viruses causes respiratory (and other) illnesses that specific vaccines are unlikely to be successful.

In the microbiology laboratories, work will become increasingly technological, with increasing attention paid to the biochemistry of the organisms and to the testing of bacteria for resistance. Microbiologists are already to be seen outside their laboratories and in the wards, being involved more and more with the actual treatment of patients. With increasing student interest in the subject, microbiology will regain a place in the medical curriculum which to some extent it had lost, as for a time it seemed that infectious disease — as a substantial threat to western man — had been beaten.

There is nothing easy or (necessarily) cheap about infection control, and real threats to its success are a lack of adequate funds, complacency and laziness. Further, perhaps the main single challenge to those concerned with the control of infection in the future is to ensure that what we already know is used effectively. We know now, without further research, how to combat the diseases which are still killing people in the developing world in their millions, sending thousands of babies to a premature grave, and reducing the vitality of farmers and breadwinners to an extent that prevents them contributing properly to the wellbeing of their families and their nations. It is not a matter of scientific knowledge. It is a matter of political and personal will.

Appendix A:
Sources

Abbott, J.D. and Robertson, L., The isolation of salmonellas from minced meat: a report from the Public Health Laboratory Service Salmonella Subcommittee, *Environmental Health*, 1980, 88:123.

Adler, M.W., *ABC of AIDS*, British Medical Journal, London, 1987.

Advisory Committee on Dangerous Pathogens, *Acquired Immune Deficiency Syndrome (AIDS) Interim Guidelines*, Health and Safety Executive and the Health Departments of the United Kingdom, 1984.

Alcock, P.A. *Food Poisoning*, Lewis, London, 1983.

Anderson, R. and May, R., The logic of vaccination, *New Scientist* 1982, 96:410.

Benenson, A.S., *Control of Communicable Diseases in Man*, 14th Edition, American Public Health Association, Washington D.C., 1985.

Blumberg, B.S., Sutnick, A.I. and London, W.T., Hepatitis and leukemia: their relation to Australia antigen, *Bulletin of the New York Academy of Medicine* 1968, 44:1566.

British Dental Association, *Guide to Blood Borne Viruses and the Control of Cross Infection in Dentistry*, London, 1987.

British Medical Association, *Deprivation and Ill-health*, Discussion Paper of the Board of Science and Education, London, 1987.

British Medical Association, *Immunisation Against Hepatitis B*, Report of Board of Science and Education, 1987.

Burnet, M. and White, D.O., *Natural History of Infectious Disease*, 4th Edition, Cambridge University Press, Cambridge, 1972.

Burton, L.E. and Smith, H.H., *Public Health and Community Medicine for the Allied Medical Professions*, 2nd Edition, Williams and Wilkins, Baltimore, 1975.

Centers for Disease Control, Mumps vaccine, *Morbidity and Mortality Weekly Report*, 1982, 31:617.

Central Statistical Office, *Social Trends 18, 1988 Edition*, HMSO, London, 1988.

Chadwick, E., *Report on the Sanitary Conditions of the Labouring Population of Great Britain*, HMSO, London, 1842.

Christie, A.B., *Infectious Diseases: Epidemiology and Clinical Practice*, 3rd Edition, Churchill Livingstone, Edinburgh, 1980.

Creighton, C., *A History of Epidemics in Britain, 1894*, 2nd Edition, with additional material by Eversley, D.E.C. *et al.*, Cambridge University Press, Cambridge, 1965.

Dawood, R., *Travellers' Health*, Oxford University Press, Oxford, 1987.

Department of Health and Social Security and the Welsh Office, *Typhoid and Paratyphoid Fevers*, HMSO, London, 1972.

Department of Health and Social Security, *On the State of the Public Health*, Annual Report of the Chief Medical Officer of the DHSS for the year 1986, HMSO, London, 1987.

Fraser, D.W. *et al.*, Legionnaires disease: description of an epidemic of pneumonia, *New England Journal of Medicine* 1977, 297:1189.

Gruneberg, R.N. (editor), *Antibiotics and Chemotherapy: Current Topics*, MTP Press, Lancaster, 1980.

Gruneberg, R.N., *Microbiology for Clinicians*, MTP Press, Lancaster, 1981.

Hepner, E., Food poisoning and salmonella infections in England and Wales 1973–75, *Public Health (London)* 1980, 94:337.

Hobbs, B.C., and Gilbert, R.J., *Food Poisoning and Food Hygiene*, 4th Edition, Edward Arnold, London, 1978.

Howe, G.M., *Man, Environment and Disease in Britain*, David and Charles, Newton Abbot, 1972.

Joint Commission on Vaccination and Immunisation, *Immunisation Against Infectious Disease*, Department of Health and Social Security, Scottish Home and Health Department and Welsh Office, London, 1984.

Knight, R., *Parasitic Disease in Man*, Churchill Livingstone, Edinburgh, 1982.

Leading Article, Failure to Vaccinate, *Lancet* 1983, 2:1343.

Lowbury, E.J.L. *et al.*, *Control of Hospital Infection*, 2nd Edition, Chapman and Hall, London, 1981.

Lucas, A.O. and Gilles, H.M., *A Short Textbook of Preventive Medicine for the Tropics*, 2nd Edition, Hodder and Stoughton, London, 1984.

Mann, J., AIDS, *World Health Forum* 1987, 8:361.

McKeown, T., *The Role of Medicine: Dream, Mirage or Nemesis?*, Nuffield Provincial Hospitals Trust, London, 1976.

Medical Research Council, National survey of tuberculosis notifications in England and Wales 1978–79, *British Medical Journal* 1980, 281:895.

Nightingale, F., *Notes on Nursing: what it is and what it is not*. Duckworth Press, London, 1952.

Office of Population Censuses and Surveys, Communicable Disease Surveillance Centre of the Public Health Laboratory Service, *Communicable Disease Statistics, 1985 Statistical Tables*, Series MB2 no. 12, HMSO, London, 1987.

Palmer, A.W., *The Penguin Dictionary of Modern History*, Penguin, 1962.

Parry, W.H., *Communicable Diseases: An Epidemiological Approach*, 2nd Edition, The English Universities Press, London, 1973.

Reid, D., Grist, N.R. and Pinkerton, I.W., *Infections in Current Medical Practice*, Update Publications, London, 1986.

Reid, D. *et al.*, Infection and travel: the experience of package tourists and other travellers, *Journal of Infection* 1980, 2:365.

Reid, D., Grist, N.R. and Najera R., Illness associated with 'package tours': a combined Spanish–Scottish study, *Bulletin of the World Health Organisation* 1978, 56:117.

Rogers, R. and Salvage, J., *Nurses at Risk: A Guide to Health and Safety at Work*, Heinemann Press, London, 1988.

Royal College of Nursing, *Introduction to Hepatitis B and Nursing Guidelines for Infection Control*, London, 1987.

Royal Society of Medicine, *Family Medical Guide*, Royal Society of Medicine, 1980.

Shanson, D.C., *Microbiology in Clinical Practice*, Wright, Bristol, 1982.

Sharp, J.C.M. and Collier, P.W., Food poisoning in Scotland, *Journal of Infection* 1981, 3:286.

Spink, W.W., *Infectious Diseases: Prevention and Treatment in the Nineteenth and Twentieth Centuries*, Dawson, Folkestone, 1978.

Truswell, A.S., *ABC of Nutrition*, British Medical Journal, London, 1986.

Tyrrell, D.A.J., *The Abolition of Infection: Hope or Illusion?*, Nuffield Provincial Hospitals Trust, London, 1982.

Walker, E. and Williams, G., *ABC of Healthy Travel*, British Medical Journal, London, 1985.

Walker, W., The Aberdeen typhoid outbreak of 1964, *Scottish Medical Journal* 1965, 10:466.

Wilson, C. and Manson-Bahr, P.E., *Manson's Tropical Diseases*, Baillière Tindall, London, 1972.

Wilson, G.J. and Miles, A.A., *Topley and Wilson's Principles and Practice of Bacteriology, Virology and Immunity*, 6th Edition, Edward Arnold, London, 1975.

World Health Forum, Smallpox eradication, a WHO success story, *World Health Forum* 1987, 8:283.

World Health Organisation, *Human Viruses in Water, Wastewater and Soil*, Technical Report Series 639, WHO, Geneva, 1979.

World Health Organisation, *Viral Respiratory Diseases*, Technical Report Series 642, WHO, Geneva, 1980.

World Health Organisation, *Environmental Management for Vector Control*, Technical Report Series 649, WHO, Geneva, 1980.

World Health Organisation, *The Leishmaniases*, Technical Report Series 701, WHO, Geneva, 1984.

World Health Organisation, *WHO Expert Committee on Rabies, Seventh Report*, Technical Report Series 709, WHO, Geneva, 1984.

World Health Organisation, *Arthropod-borne and Rodent-borne Viral Diseases*, Technical Report Series 719, WHO, Geneva, 1985.

World Health Organisation, *Viral Haemorrhagic Fevers*, Technical Report Series 721, WHO, Geneva, 1985.

World Health Organisation, *WHO Expert Committee on Malaria, Eighteenth Report*, Technical Report Series 735, WHO, Geneva, 1986.

World Health Organisation, *WHO Expert Committee on Venereal Diseases and Treponematoses, Sixth Report*, Technical Report Series 736, WHO, Geneva, 1986.

World Health Organisation, *Joint FAO/WHO Expert Committee on Brucellosis, Sixth Report*, Technical Report Series 740, WHO, Geneva, 1986.

World Health Organisation, *Technology for Water Supply and Sanitation in Developing Countries*, Technical Report Series 742, WHO, Geneva, 1987.

World Health Organisation, *Prevention and Control of Intestinal Parasitic Infections*, Technical Report Series 749, WHO, Geneva, 1987.

World Health Organisation, *Progress in the Development and Use of Antiviral Drugs and Interferon*, Technical Report Series 754, WHO, Geneva, 1987.

World Health Organisation, Cardiovascular diseases in developed world, respiratory diseases in developing, *World Health* 1984, August/September:30.

World Health Organisation, *Vaccination Requirements and Health Advice for International Travel, Situation as on 1 January 1988*, WHO, Geneva, 1988.

Yekutiel, P., *Eradication of Infectious Diseases: A Critical Study*, Contributions to Epidemiology and Biostatistics, Volume 2, Karger, Basle, 1980.

Youmans, G.P., Paterson, P.Y. and Sommers, H.M., *The Biological and Clinical Basis of Infectious Diseases*, 2nd Edition, Saunders, Philadelphia, 1980.

Appendix B: Some Important Organisms

The more important organisms are listed in this appendix, together with a note on the sites where they are most customarily found, the diseases for which they are mainly responsible, and the therapeutic agents and drugs most commonly used to treat these diseases. The list is, of course, far from being entirely comprehensive, and for more information on specific organisms, diseases and treatment standard texts (such as those cited in Appendix A) should be consulted.

ORGANISMS AND USUAL SOURCES	TYPICAL DISEASES	TYPICAL THERAPEUTIC AGENTS
Cocci		
Staphylococcus		
S. aureus Common in the noses and sometimes on the skins of healthy people; common cause of infection, especially in hospitals; spread from person to person	Skin infections such as boils and carbuncles; infections of internal organs and tissues including bones and joints; blood poisoning; toxins commonly cause food poisoning, rarely toxic shock (e.g. from tampons)	Penicillin (often resistant); cloxacillin; erythromycin; lincomycin; fusidic acid; vancomycin
S. epidermidis or *S. albus* In noses and on skins of healthy people	Usually not pathogenic, but may cause infection in hospitals	Varied; hospital infections will need sensitivity testing

Streptococcus

S. pneumoniae, or pneumococci In noses and throats of most people	Infections of the middle ear and sinuses; pneumonia; meningitis	Penicillin; erythromycin
S. viridans Normal inhabitants of upper respiratory tract and intestine	Inflammation of the lining of the heart and heart valves; abscesses of internal organs	Penicillin; erythromycin
S. pyogenes **Group A** In upper respiratory tract of small proportion of people	Sore throats, scarlet fever, ear infections; as severe complication of other conditions—rheumatic fever, wound infection, puerperal sepsis, blood poisoning	Penicillin; erythromycin
Group B In vagina and on perineal skin	Infection of the newborn, including meningitis and blood poisoning	Erythromycin; penicillin
Groups C and G In the throat	Rare cause of sore throats, wound and blood infections	Penicillin; erythromycin
S. faecalis, or enterococci In intestine	Infections of the urinary tract and heart lining	Erythromycin; penicillin

Neisseria

N. meningitidis, or meningococcus In the nose and throat of up to one-third of all people	Important cause of meningitis in Britain, especially in children	Penicillin
N. gonorrhoea, or gonococcus Found in urinary and genital tracts of infected people	Gonorrhoea; eye infection of newborn during birth	Penicillin; spectinomycin for resistant strains

Bacilli

Bacillus

B. anthracis Spores live in soil	Anthrax (a zoonosis)	Penicillin
B. cereus In soil, air	Toxins cause food poisoning (contaminates boiled rice)	Fluid replacement

Corynebacterium

C. diphtheriae Rarely found in normal throat; related 'diphtheroids' are not pathogenic and are commonly found in throat and on skin	The toxin of some strains causes diphtheria	Penicillin; erythromycin; prevented by toxoid

Clostridium

C. perfringens, or welchii

In soil and on dirty skin, and in faeces of healthy people

Gas gangrene following contamination of wound; food poisoning

Penicillin

C. tetani

Common in soil and animal faeces

Tetanus ('lockjaw')

Immunoglobulin and penicillin; prevented by toxoid

Escherichia

E. coli, one of the 'coliforms', or enterobacteria

Abundant in normal human intestine; normally not a pathogen

Gastroenteritis; urinary tract infections; wound infections

Ampicillin; co-trimoxazole; but such treatment depending on sensitivity

Klebsiella

Klebsiella species are widely distributed in the natural environment

Hospital infections

Gentamicin; cephalosporins; but will depend on strain

Salmonella

S. typhimurium is one of more than 1,500 types that cause food poisoning; common in intestines of many animals and birds, especially poultry

Food poisoning ('acute gastroenteritis')

Fluid replacement; antibiotics rarely necessary

S. typhi, paratyphi A, paratyphi B

Found in faeces of carriers

Typhoid fever (enteric fever) and paratyphoid fever

Chloramphenicol; or other antibiotics depending on sensitivity

Shigella

S. dysenteriae, flexneri, boydii, sonnei

In faeces of infected people

Shigellosis (dysentery)

Fluid replacement; antibiotics depending on sensitivity

Pseudomonas

P. aeruginosa

In intestines of animals and humans (especially patients treated with antibiotics in hospital); survives and multiplies anywhere moist in hospital environment

Important cause of hospital infections, especially of the urinary tract, skin, ears, respiratory tract, burns, wounds

Aminoglycosides (e.g. streptomycin, gentamicin, tobramycin); some penicillins depending on strain

Vibrios

V. cholerae

In faeces of infected people; can persist in water and in seafood

Cholera

Fluid replacement; tetracycline

Campylobacter jejuni, coli In faeces of animals and infants	Important cause of diarrhoeal disease, especially infants and travellers	Fluids; antibiotics for prolonged cases

Parvobacteria

Haemophilus influenzae and other species Common in normal throat	Infections in young children, e.g. respiratory, meningitis, osteomyelitis; contributes to chronic bronchitis in adults	Ampicillin (but many strains now resistant); chloramphenicol; co-trimoxazole; tetracycline
Bordetella pertussis In throats of infected people	Whooping cough (pertussis)	Prevented by vaccine; antibiotics have little effect on symptoms
Legionella pneumophila Found in water, e.g. hot and cold water taps and showers, air-conditioning towers, creeks and ponds; moist soil	Legionellosis (Legionnaires' disease), a form of pneumonia	Erythromycin; plus rifampicin in severe cases; tetracycline
Yersinia pestis Wild rodents	Plague	Streptomycin; tetracycline; chloramphenicol
Brucella species Milk and cheese from infected cattle, pigs, goats and sheep	Brucellosis	Tetracycline plus streptomycin; co-trimoxazole; rifampicin

Mycobacterium

M. tuberculosis, bovis Infected sputum	Tuberculosis; bovine tuberculosis (a zoonosis)	Isoniazid, with rifampicin, streptomycin, ethambutol and pyrazinamide in various combinations

Spirochaetes

Treponema pallidum Infected body fluids	Syphilis	Penicillin; tetracycline; erythromycin
Treponema pertenue Skin of infected people	Yaws	Penicillin
Leptospira icterohaemorrhagiae, hebdomadis, canicola	Leptospirosis (a zoonosis)	Penicillin in high doses; doxycycline
Borrelia burgdorferi	Lyme disease (a zoonosis)	Tetracycline; penicillin

Chlamydiae

C. trachomatis In infected body fluids	Trachoma; genital infections; conjunctivitis; infant pneumonia; lymphogranuloma venereum	Tetracycline; doxycycline; erythromycin
C. psittaci	Psittacosis (a zoonosis)	Tetracycline group

Rickettsiae

Rickettsia prowazeki Carried by lice	Typhus fever	Doxycycline; tetracycline; chloramphenicol

Other rickettsiae Carried by ticks	Rocky Mountain spotted fever, tick fevers and various forms of tick typhus named by place of origin	Tetracycline group; chloramphenicol
Coxiella burnetii Infected sheep and cattle	Q fever	Tetracycline; chloramphenicol

Mycoplasmas

M. pneumoniae In nose and throat	Lower respiratory infection; pneumonia	Erythromycin; tetracycline

Viruses

Respiratory viruses

Influenza A, B, C	Influenza	Vaccines available; amantadine helps prevention
Rhinoviruses	Colds	None specific
Adenoviruses	Respiratory infection; conjunctivitis	None specific
Paramyxoviruses	Mumps; measles; respiratory syncytial syndrome in infants	Vaccines available; no specific treatment
Epstein-Barr virus	Infectious mononucleosis (glandular fever)	None specific; steroids may help severe cases

Enteroviruses

Polio viruses	Poliomyelitis	Vaccines available
Coxsackie viruses	Respiratory, nervous system and heart infections	None specific
Echoviruses	Respiratory, nervous system and intestinal infections	None specific
Rotavirus	Severe gastroenteritis of infants and young children	Fluid replacement; none specific
Hepatitis A virus	Hepatitis A (infectious hepatitis, epidemic jaundice)	None specific

Herpes viruses

Herpes simplex virus (HSV)	HSV type 1 causes herpes sores of lips and face, rare infection of the nervous system; type 2, genital herpes	Some antiviral drugs helpful, e.g. idoxuridine, acyclovir
Varicella-zoster	Chickenpox and shingles	Vidarabine, acyclovir in immune deficiency; immune globulin
Cytomegalovirus	Neonatal infection	None specific

Blood-borne viruses

Human immunodeficiency virus (HIV)	Acquired immune deficiency syndrome (AIDS)	None specific (see text)
Hepatitis B virus	Hepatitis B (serum hepatitis)	Vaccine available; no specific treatment

Arthopod-borne viruses; zoonoses

Arboviruses	Various forms of encephalitis; yellow fever; dengue; haemorrhagic fevers	Vaccine for yellow fever; no specific drug treatment
Arenaviruses	Lassa fever; meningitis	None specific
Rabies virus	Rabies	Vaccine available

Other viruses

Pox viruses	Smallpox (previously); monkeypox; vaccinia; dermatitis	Smallpox vaccine no longer required; no specific drug treatment for others
Rubella virus	Rubella (German measles)	Vaccine available for groups at risk
Coronaviruses	Upper respiratory infections	None specific

Protozoa

Entamoeba histolytica Contaminated water	Amoebic dysentery; liver abscess	Metronidazole; diloxanide
Giardia lamblia Human faeces	Diarrhoea (giardiasis)	Metronidazole; chloroquine; mepacrine
Plasmodium vivax, malariae, falciparum and *ovale* Transmitted by mosquito	Malaria	Prevented by chloroquine or other drugs depending on local resistance; treated with chloroquine, amodiaquine, quinine
Leishmania tropica and other species Animal reservoirs; transmitted by sandflies	Leishmaniasis (skin sores and ulcers; kala azar)	Sodium stibogluconate
Trypanosoma brucei Transmitted by tsetse fly and triatoma bug	Sleeping sickness; African and South American forms	Suramin; pentamidine
Toxoplasma gondii Cat faeces and raw meat	Toxoplasmosis	Pyrimethamine and sulphonamide

Helminths

Enterobius vermicularis Contaminated fomites	Threadworms (pinworms)	Piperazine; thiabendazole; mebendazole

Ascaris lumbricoides Soil	Roundworms	Piperazine; thiabendazole; mebendazole
Taenia, Diphyllobothrium and *Hymenolepsis* species Raw or poorly cooked meat and fish	Tapeworms	Niclosamide
Ancylostoma and *Necator* species Faeces in soil	Hookworms	Tetrachloroethylene; bephenium; pyrantel
Schistosoma species Infested water	Schistosomiasis (bilharziasis)	Praziquantel; oxamniquine; metriphonate
Wuchereria bancrofti, Onchocerca species, and *Brugia* species Transmitted by mosquitos	Filariasis ('elephantiasis')	Diethylcarbamazine
Strongyloides stercoralis Faeces in soil	Strongyloidiasis (threadworms)	Thiabendazole
Trichinella spiralis Infected poorly cooked pork	Trichiniasis (trichinosis, pork roundworm)	Mebendazole
Echinococcus granulosus Dog faeces	Hydatid disease (dog tapeworm)	Mebendazole may be effective

Fungi

Superficial mycoses

Microsporum, Trichophyton and *Epidermophyton* species	Tinea (ringworm) of skin, nails and hair	Griseofulvin; ketoconazole; clotrimazole; econazole; miconazole
Aspergillus niger	External ear infection	Non-specific
Candida albicans	Thrush, monilial vaginitis, skin and nail infection	Clotrimazole; econazole; miconazole; nystatin

Deep mycoses

Candida albicans and many other fungi	Chest, kidney, blood and heart infection, especially in immune deficiency states	Amphotericin; flucytosine

Index